HPNA PALLIATIVE NURSING MANUALS

Spiritual, Religious, and Cultural Aspects of Care

Edited by

Betty R. Ferrell, RN, PhD, MA, FAAN, FPCN, CHPN

Professor and Director
Department of Nursing Research and Education
City of Hope Comprehensive Cancer Center
Duarte, California

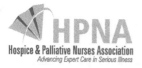

Hospice & Palliative Nurses Association
Advancing Expert Care in Serious Illness

OXFORD
UNIVERSITY PRESS

OXFORD

UNIVERSITY PRESS

Oxford University Press is a department of the University of
Oxford. It furthers the University's objective of excellence in research,
scholarship, and education by publishing worldwide.

Oxford   New York
Auckland   Cape Town   Dar es Salaam   Hong Kong   Karachi
Kuala Lumpur   Madrid   Melbourne   Mexico City   Nairobi
New Delhi   Shanghai   Taipei   Toronto

With offices in
Argentina   Austria   Brazil   Chile   Czech Republic   France   Greece
Guatemala   Hungary   Italy   Japan   Poland   Portugal   Singapore
South Korea   Switzerland   Thailand   Turkey   Ukraine   Vietnam

Oxford is a registered trademark of Oxford University Press
in the UK and certain other countries.

Published in the United States of America by
Oxford University Press
198 Madison Avenue, New York, NY 10016

© Oxford University Press 2016

Library of Congress Cataloging-in-Publication Data
Spiritual, religious, and cultural aspects of care/edited by Betty R. Ferrell.
p. ; cm.
(HPNA palliative nursing manuals ; volume 5)
Includes bibliographical references and index.
ISBN 978–0–19–024423–1 (alk. paper)
I. Ferrell, Betty, editor.   II. Hospice and Palliative Nurses Association, issuing body.
III. Series: HPNA palliative nursing manuals ; v. 5.
[DNLM: 1. Hospice and Palliative Care Nursing.   2. Spirituality.   3. Culturally Competent Care.
4. Palliative Care.   5. Pastoral Care.   6. Terminal Care. WY 152.3]
RT87.T45
616.02′9—dc23
2015009169

9 8 7 6 5 4 3
Printed in Canada

Contents

>

Preface

This is the fifth volume of a series being published by Oxford University Press in collaboration with the Hospice and Palliative Nurses Association. The intent of this series is to provide palliative care nurses with quick reference guides to each of the key domains of palliative care.

Content for this series was derived primarily from the *Oxford Textbook of Palliative Nursing* (4th edition, 2015) which is edited by Betty Ferrell, the editor of this series, Nessa Coyle, and Judith Paice. The Contributors identified in each volume are the authors of chapters in the *Oxford Textbook of Palliative Nursing* from which the content was selected for this volume. The Textbook contains more extensive content and references, so users of this Palliative Nursing Series are encouraged to use the Textbook as an additional resource.

This volume presents key content on the vital topics of spiritual, cultural, and existential aspects of serious illness. Providing true, patient-centered palliative care means addressing all aspects of quality of life, including spiritual care. Nurses increasingly care for patients and families from diverse cultures and for those with deep existential concerns, as they face life-threatening disease or the end of life. The intent of this volume is to support nurses in improving this essential aspect of palliative care.

Betty R. Ferrell, RN, PhD, MA, FAAN, FPCN, CHPN

Contributors

Rev. Pamela Baird, AS
End-of-Life Practitioner
Seasons of Life
Arcadia, California

Tami Borneman, RN, MSN, CNS, FPCN
Senior Research Specialist
Nursing Research and Education
City of Hope National
   Medical Center
Duarte, California

Katherine Brown-Saltzman, RN, MA
Clinical Specialist in Palliative Care
UCLA Medical Center
Los Angeles, California

Valerie T. Cotter, DrNP, AGPCNP-BC, FAANP
Advanced Senior Lecturer
Director of Adult-Gerontology
   Primary Care Nurse Practitioner
   Program
University of Pennsylvania School
   of Nursing
Philadelphia, Pennsylvania

Anessa M. Foxwell, MSN, CRNP
Palliative Care Service
Hospital of the University
   of Pennsylvania
Philadelphia, Pennsylvania

Elizabeth Johnston Taylor, PhD, RN
Associate Professor, School
   of Nursing
Loma Linda University
Loma Linda, California

Polly Mazanec, PhD, ACNP-BC, AOCN, FPCN
Assistant Professor of Nursing
Case Western Reserve University
Cleveland, Ohio

Joan T. Panke, MA, APN, ACHPN
Palliative Consultant/Palliative
   Care NP
Arlington, Virginia

Chapter 1

Spiritual Assessment

Elizabeth Johnston Taylor

To solve any problem, one must first assess what the problem is. Consequently, the nursing process dictates that the nurse begins care with an assessment of the patient's health needs. Although palliative nurses assess patients' pain experiences, hydration status, and medical issues, they assess less frequently patients' and family members' spirituality.

Because spirituality is an inherent, integrating, and often extremely valued dimension for those who receive palliative nursing care, it is essential that palliative care nurses know how to conduct a spiritual assessment. This chapter reviews spiritual assessment models, presents general guidelines on how to conduct a spiritual assessment, and discusses what the nurse ought to do with spiritual assessment data. These topics are prefaced by arguments supporting the need for spiritual assessments, descriptions of what spirituality "looks like" among the terminally ill, and risk factors for those who are likely to experience spiritual distress. But first, a description of spirituality is in order.

What Is Spirituality?

Numerous analyses of spirituality have identified key aspects of this ethereal and intangible phenomenon. Conceptualizations of spirituality often include the need for purpose and meaning, forgiveness, love and relatedness, hope, creativity, and religious faith and its expression. A classic nursing definition for spirituality authored by Reed[1] proposed that spirituality involves meaning-making through intrapersonal, interpersonal, and transpersonal connection. More recent spirituality definitions accepted by healthcare scholars not only emphasize the human search for ultimate meaning, but also the human desire for harmonious connectedness with self, others, an ultimate Other, and for some, the environment.[2]

Usually, spirituality is differentiated from religion—the organized, codified, and often institutionalized beliefs and practices that express one's spirituality.[3] To use Narayansamy's[4] metaphor: "Spirituality is more of a journey and religion may be the transport to help us in our journey" (p. 141). Definitions of spirituality include transcendence—that is, spirituality explains the need to transcend the self, manifested in a recognition of an Ultimate Other, Sacred Source, Higher Power, divinity, or God. Although these definitions allow for an open interpretation of what a person considers to be sacred or transcendent, some have argued that such a definition is inappropriate for atheists, humanists, and those who do not accept a spiritual reality.[5] Indeed, a pluralistic definition of spirituality (however "elastic" and vague it is) is necessary for ethical practice, and a spiritual assessment process that is sensitive to the myriad of worldviews is essential—if even appropriate for those who reject a spiritual reality.[6]

The spiritual assessment methods introduced in this chapter are influenced by some conceptualization of spirituality. Some, however, have questioned whether spiritual assessment is possible, given the broad, encompassing definition typically espoused by nurses.[7,8] Bash contended that spirituality is an "elastic" term that cannot be universally defined. Because a patient's definition of spirituality may differ from the nurse's assumptions about it, Bash argued that widely applicable tools for spiritual assessment are impossible to design. It is important to note that the literature and methods for spiritual assessment presented in this chapter are primarily from the United States and United Kingdom, influenced most by Western Judeo-Christian traditions and peoples. Hence, they are most applicable to these people.

Why Is It Important for a Palliative Care Nurse to Conduct a Spiritual Assessment?

Spiritual awareness increases as one faces an imminent death.[9,10] Although some may experience spiritual distress or "soul pain," others may have a spiritual transformation or experience spiritual growth and health. There is mounting empirical evidence to suggest that persons with terminal illnesses consider spirituality to be one of the most important contributors to quality of life.[11] Research findings from various studies indicate that spiritual well-being may protect terminal cancer patients against end of life despair; it also has moderately strong inverse relationships with the desire for a hastened death, hopelessness, and suicidal ideations. Religious beliefs and practices (e.g., prayer, beliefs that explain suffering or death) are valued and frequently used as helpful coping strategies by those who suffer and die from physical illness.[3] Family caregivers of seriously ill patients find comfort and strength from their spirituality that assists them in coping.[12,13]

These research themes imply that attention to the spirituality of terminally ill patients and their caregivers is of utmost importance. That is, if patients' spiritual resources assist them in coping, and if imminent death precipitates heightened spiritual awareness and concerns, and if patients view their spiritual health as most important to their quality of life, then spiritual assessment that initiates a process promoting spiritual health is vital to effective palliative care. It is for these reasons that the National Consensus Project (NCP) and National Quality Forum included guidelines and preferred practices for supporting spirituality in palliative care.[14] The NCP guidelines (5.1) state: "Spiritual and existential dimensions are assessed and responded to, based upon the best available evidence, which is skillfully and systematically applied."

The Joint Commission has mandated a spiritual assessment be included in palliative care.[15] It stipulates that for clients entering an approved facility, a spiritual assessment should, at least, "determine the patient's denomination, beliefs, and what spiritual practices are important." They also require that the institution define the scope and process of the assessment, and specify who completes it. Often, it is nurses who are charged with completing the spiritual assessment as part of an intake assessment.

Why should palliative care nurses be conducting spiritual assessments? After all, chaplains and clergy are the trained spiritual care experts. That said, although chaplains are the trained experts in spiritual care, current main-stream thinking asserts that all hospice team members participate in spiritual caregiving. A multidisciplinary consensus project offered the following guide-lines for spiritual care at end of life:

- Upon admission, all patients should be screened for spiritual distress, and a referral made if support is needed.
- Structured assessment tools should be used to document and evaluate care.
- All palliative care clinicians should be trained to recognize and report spiritual distress.
- All clinicians should be trained to spiritually screen, and a certified chaplain should complete a more thorough assessment.
- Screenings and assessments should be documented.
- Patients should be re-assessed, when their condition changes.[16]

Not only do professional palliative care recommendations include nurses in the spiritual assessment process, but there are also generic nursing ethics and professional standards that support the nurse's role in health-related spiritual and religious assessment.[3] Indeed, considering nurses' frontline position, coordination role, and intimacy with patients' concerns, the holistic perspective on care, and even lack of religious cloaking, nurses can be the ideal professionals to perform an initial spiritual assessment, if properly prepared.

Nurses must recognize, however, that they are not specialists in spiritual assessment and caregiving; they are generalists. Most oncology and hospice nurses report they lack adequate training in spiritual assessment and care; in fact, it is this absence of training, accompanied by role confusion, lack of time, and other factors that nurses often cite as barriers to completing spiritual assessments.[17,18] Therefore, when a nurse's assessment indicates need for further sensitive assessment and specialized care, it is imperative that a referral to a spiritual care specialist (e.g., chaplain, clergy, patient's spiritual director) be made.

How Does Spirituality Manifest Itself?

To understand how to assess spirituality, the palliative care nurse must know what subjective and objective observations indicate spiritual distress or well-being. Numerous descriptive studies have identified the spiritual needs of patients and their loved ones facing the end of life.[19] Likewise, clinicians have written articles that describe the spiritual concerns of these persons. Box 1.1 provides a fairly comprehensive listing of end of life spiritual needs compiled by Puchalski and colleagues.[2]

Box 1.1 End of Life Spiritual Needs

- Lack of meaning and purpose (e.g., "Why do I have to suffer on the way to death? Why couldn't I just go to my death in my sleep?" [meaningless- ness of suffering]; "I feel like I never really did anything important in life, and now it's too late.")
- Despair and hopelessness (e.g., "I just want to give up . . . its not worth it anymore" [although some would argue that complete hopelessness is incompatible with life, hopefulness is sometimes hard to feel].)
- Religious struggle (e.g., "Sometimes it is hard to believe there is a loving God upstairs that has my best interests in mind" [religious struggles can arise for those who have not been religious during their adulthood, as they may struggle with the beliefs instilled in them dur- ing childhood].)
- Not being remembered (e.g., "Death is just so final; I know my friends will eventually move on and I'll have been like a blip on the monitor.")
- Guilt and shame (e.g., "I think my cancer is a punishment for something I did when I was young.")
- Loss of dignity (e.g., "Look and smell this body! It's so embarrassing . . . it's not me anymore.")
- Lack of love, loneliness (e.g., "Everyone is so busy. . . . too busy to take care of me.")
- Anger at God/others (e.g., "Why would a loving God allow this to hap- pen to me?")
- Perceiving abandonment by God/others (e.g., "I feel like my prayers aren't being answered . . . where is God?")
- Feeling out of control (e.g., "I'm ready to go . . . but it's not happening.")
- Distress secondary to misinterpretation of religious dogma or religious or spiritual community actions that impede full development of human potential
- Reconciliation (e.g., desire to be reunited with estranged family members)
- Grief/loss (spiritual issues often accompany the various losses persons mourn when living with a terminal illness, such as the loss of indepen- dence, social roles and vocation, body image and function)
- Gratitude (e.g., "Now I have learned to appreciate the little things in life, and I'm just so happy for each new day that dawns.")

Although the term *spiritual needs* may suggest a problem, they also can be of a positive nature. For example, patients can have a need to express their joy about sensing closeness to others, or to pursue activities that allow expression of creative impulses (e.g., creating artwork, music making, writing). The following models for conducting a spiritual assessment will provide fur- ther understanding of how spirituality manifests.

Spiritual Assessment Models

Although some assessment models have been published during the past few years, many were developed in the 1990s, when the research about spiritual care began to proliferate. Some were developed by clinicians caring for the terminally ill, while others—easily adapted or used with those at the end of life—were developed for general use for those with an illness.

Many advocate a two-tiered approach to spiritual assessment. The first tier, a brief assessment for screening purposes, is conducted when a patient enters a healthcare institution for palliative care.[2,3,20] If this assessment reveals there are spiritual needs, then spiritual care can only be planned if further information is collected. The second assessment tier allows for focused, in-depth assessment. Some chaplains distinguish a spiritual assessment from a spiritual history, an in-depth review of one's spiritual journey through life (best done by a trained chaplain or spiritual care expert). After this chapter reviews recommended spiritual screening questions, it presents more comprehensive models or approaches.

Screening

While recognizing society's spiritual plurality, and that some may not experience a spiritual reality, an initial screening must assess a patient's basic orientation.[3] Others assume spirituality is universal and suggest that a spiritual screening check for the significance of the beliefs and practices to the present illness, and ascertain how the patient may want spiritual support from the healthcare team. Various clinical authors suggest using single questions to broach spirituality with a patient. For example:

- How important is spirituality or religion to you?[21] Kub and colleagues,[22] in their research with 114 terminally ill persons, found that a single question about the importance of religion reveals far more than a question about frequency of religious service attendance—a question that has often been the sole spiritual assessment in some institutions.
- What do you rely on in times of illness?[23]
- Are you at peace? This question was found to correlate highly with spiritual and emotional well-being in a large study of terminally ill patients.[24]

Two concise screening approaches have been proposed by physicians Lo and colleagues[25] for use in palliative care settings:

- Is faith/religion/spirituality important to you in this illness? Has faith been important to you at other times in your life?
- Do you have someone to talk to about religious matters? Would you like to explore religious matters with someone?

Striving to have an even more streamlined spiritual assessment, Matthews and colleagues[26] suggested that initial spiritual assessments be limited to asking, "Is your religion [or faith] helpful to you in handling your illness?" and "What can I do to support your faith or religious commitment?"

Several clinicians have devised mnemonic tools for use in spiritual assessment (see Table 1.1). Although some of these are fairly comprehensive,

Table 1.1 Mnemonics to Guide a Spiritual Assessment

Author/s	Components (Mnemonic)	Illustrative Questions
Maugens[49]	• S (spiritual belief system)	What is your formal religious affiliation?
	• P (personal spirituality)	Describe the beliefs and practices of your religion or spiritual system that you personally accept. What is the importance of your spirituality/religion in daily life?
	• I (integration with a spiritual community)	Do you belong to any spiritual or religious group or community? What importance does this group have to you? Does or could this group provide help in dealing with health issues?
	• R (ritualized practices and restrictions)	Are there specific elements of medical care that you forbid on the basis of religious/spiritual grounds?
	• I (implications for medical care)	What aspects of your religion/spirituality would you like me to keep in mind as I care for you? Are there any barriers to our relationship based on religious or spiritual issues?
	• T (terminal events planning)	As we plan for your care near the end of life, how does your faith impact on your decisions?
Anandarajah & Hight[66]	• H (sources of hope)	What or who is it that gives you hope?
	• O (organized religion)	Are you a part of an organized faith group? What does this group do for you as a person?
	• P (personal spirituality or spiritual practices)	What personal spiritual practices, like prayer or meditation, help you?
	• E (effects on medical care and/or end of life issues)	Do you have any beliefs that may affect how the healthcare team cares for you?
Puchalski[27]	• F (faith)	Do you have a faith belief? What is it that gives your life meaning?
	• I (import or Influence)	What importance does your faith have in your life? How does your faith belief influence your life?
	• C (community)	Are you a member of a faith community? How does this support you?
	• A (address)	How would you like for me to integrate or address these issues in your care?
LaRocca-Pitts[67]	• F (faith)	What spiritual beliefs are important to you now?
	• A (availability/ accessibility/applicability)	Are you able to find the spiritual nurture that you would like now?

(continued)

Table 1.1 (Continued)

Author/s	Components (Mnemonic)	Illustrative Questions
	• C (coping/comfort)	How comforting/helpful are your spiritual beliefs at this time?
	• T (treatment)	How can I/we provide spiritual support?
Skalla & McCoy[50]	• M (moral authority)	Where does your sense of what to do come from? What guides you to decide what is right or wrong for you?
	• V (vocational)	What gives your life purpose? What work is important to you? What mission or role do you feel passionate about?
	• A (aesthetic)	What brings beauty or pleasure to your life now? How are you able to express your creativity? How do you deal with boredom?
	• S (social)	What people or faith community do you sense you belong with most? Do you belong to a community that nourishes you spiritually?
	• T (transcendent)	Who or what controls what happens in life? Who/what supports you when you are ill? Is there an Ultimate Other (an entity that is sacred, for example)? If so, how do you relate to It?
McEvoy (pediatric context)[68]	• B (belief system)	What religious or spiritual beliefs, if any, do members of your family have?
	• E (ethics or values)	
	• L (lifestyle)	What standards/values/rules for life does your family think important? What spiritual habits or activities does your family commit to because of spiritual beliefs? (e.g., Any sacred times to observe or diet you keep?)
	• I (involvement in spiritual community)	How connected to a faith community are you? Would you like us to help you reconnect with this group now?
	• E (education)	Are you receiving any form of religious education? How can we help you keep up with it?
	• F (near future events of spiritual significance for which to prepare the child)	Are there any upcoming religious ceremonies that you are getting ready for?

others are designed to collect superficial information—to screen. The most widely cited tool is likely Pulchaski's[27] FICA tool.

Hodge[28] essentially proposed the same content for his brief assessment, arguing that it meets The Joint Commission requirement. Hodge's assessment questions include:

- "I was wondering if spirituality or religion is important to you?
- Are there certain spiritual beliefs and practices that you find particularly helpful in dealing with problems?
- I was wondering if you attend a church or some other type of spiritual community?
- Are there any spiritual needs or concerns I can help you with?" (p. 319)

The nonintrusive tone with which these questions are worded is exemplary.

Frick and colleagues, using similar questions (i.e., "Would you describe yourself—in the broadest sense of the term—as a believing/spiritual/religious person?" "What is the place of spirituality in your life?" "How integrated are you in a spiritual community?" "What role would you like to assign to your healthcare team with regard to spirituality?"), found that these questions were helpful for both patients and physicians.[29]

Box 1.2, a prototype for a spiritual screening tool, can be adapted to any palliative care context. It can be completed by either the patient alone or with a nurse's assistance. Because it is unknown how well family can serve as proxies for spiritual health measurements, and because responses may be easily swayed by social desirability, it is best not to have family complete such a tool. Rather, the tool can be inserted in the patient chart to guide ongoing spiritual assessment and care, and is purposefully concise to accommodate the palliative care patient who is suffering from symptom distress.

Comprehensive Models

If the screening assessment or subsequent observation reveals a spiritual need that might benefit from spiritual care by a palliative care team member, then a more comprehensive assessment should follow. This more in-depth assessment of the specific spiritual need or multiple aspects of the patient's spirituality will provide the evidence upon which to plan appropriate spiritual care.[2] For example, if a nurse observes a terminally ill patient's spouse crying and stating, "Why does God have to take my sweetheart?," then the nurse would want to understand what factors are contributing to or may relieve this spiritual pain. To focus the assessment on the pertinent topic, the nurse would then ask questions that explore the spouse's "why" questions, beliefs about misfortune, perceptions of God, and spiritual coping strategies.

Criteria for a Tier 2 Spiritual Assessment

When should clinicians probe more deeply? Hodge[28] suggested four criteria for determining whether to perform a more comprehensive assessment:

- First, consider patient autonomy. The patient must give informed consent. A comprehensive assessment may drill into inner depths the patient does not wish to expose to a clinician.
- Second, consider the clinician's competency to discuss spiritual matters. Is the clinician culturally sensitive and aware of how a personal worldview might

Box 1.2 Self (or Nurse-Assisted) Spiritual Screening for Palliative Care Patients

Dear_____,

Your palliative care team wants to make sure you receive the physical, emotional, and spiritual care and comfort you need.

Typically, persons receiving palliative care find themselves becoming more aware of their spirituality or religion. Please help us to understand what are your spiritual care and comfort needs.

Directions: Place an "X" on the lines to show the answer that comes closest to describing your experience.

1. How important is spirituality and/or religion to you now?

/_____/

Not at all important   Very important

2. Recently, my spirits have been . . .

/_____/

Awful low . . . . . . okay . . . . . good . . . . . . great

What can a nurse do that would help to nurture or boost your spirits? (check all that apply)

___ pray with me

___ allow time and space for my private prayer or meditation

___ bring art or music that will nurture my spirit

___ bring or read inspiring things to me

___ listen to my thoughts about certain spiritual matters

___ provide assistance so I can record my life story

___ just be with me

___ help me to stay connected to me spiritual community by contacting:

- my church/temple/mosque/local faith community's name and location _____
- my clergy or spiritual leader's name (any contact information will be helpful) _____

Is there anything else about your spiritual beliefs or practices that the palliative care team should know about? (e.g., diet or lifestyle proscribed by your religion? beliefs guiding your preparation for death?) Please write here (or on the back side) or tell your nurse.

Reproduced by permission of Oxford University Press USA from Taylor EJ. Spiritual assessment. In: Ferrell BR, Coyle N, eds. *Oxford Textbook of Palliative Nursing*. 4th ed., New York, NY: Oxford University Press; 2015:536 (Box 32.1).

conflict with the patient's? Might the clinician suffer from religious countertransference and inappropriately relate to the patient from personal biases?

- Third, consider if the spiritual issue is relevant to the present healthcare situation. If not, it may not be in the nurse's purview. For end of life patients, however, many past and diverse spiritual struggles can resurface; although they may seem tangential to provision of present healthcare, the patient may benefit from spiritual expertise to address such issues before death.

(The nurse's curiosity or desire to evangelize the patient is never an ethical rationale for spiritual assessment.[3])

• Finally, consider the importance of spirituality to the patient. An extreme illustration: If a patient states spirituality is personally irrelevant, a comprehensive spiritual assessment would be inappropriate.

Observing these guidelines can prevent inappropriate and time-consuming assessment and care.

Although a comprehensive spiritual assessment may well be beneficial to many patients at the end of life, it is likely that few palliative care nurses are competent or able to conduct such an assessment.[2,3] Fowler posits that a person's spiritual or religious experience is arranged in layers like an onion. The outer layers of public and semipublic spiritual belief and practice are an appropriate domain for the nurse negligibly trained in spiritual assessment and care, whereas the deeper, more intimate—and often pain-filled—inner layers are best assessed and addressed by spiritual care experts.[30]

Models for Comprehensive Spiritual Assessment

The screening models presented thus far are most relevant for palliative care nurses. By reviewing more comprehensive models, however, nurses can increase their knowledge and gain appreciation for the territory that spiritual care experts may travel with patients. Nurses are in a pivotal position to refer patients to chaplains or other spiritual care specialists who can conduct a comprehensive assessment.

Fitchett,[31] a chaplain, developed the "7-by-7" model for spiritual assessment with a multidisciplinary group of health professionals. In addition to reviewing seven dimensions of a person (medical, psychological, psychosocial, family system, ethnic and cultural, societal issues, and spiritual dimensions), Fitchett suggests seven spiritual dimensions to address:

• beliefs and meaning (i.e., mission, purpose, religious and nonreligious meaning in life);

• vocation and consequences (what persons believe they should do, what their calling is);

• experience (of the divine or demonic) and emotion (the tone emerging from one's spiritual experience);

• courage and growth (the ability to encounter doubt and inner change);

• ritual and practice (activities that make life meaningful);

• community (involvement in any formal or informal community that shares spiritual beliefs and practices); and

• authority and guidance (exploring where or with whom one places trust, seeks guidance).

This model likely offers chaplains and spiritual care experts the most comprehensive approach to assessment.

Possibly the first comprehensive spiritual assessment model was that developed by Pruyser,[32] the patriarch of modern chaplaincy. Pruyser's original model identified seven aspects, each of which can be viewed as a continuum. These aspects of spirituality included:

- awareness of the holy, or the lack thereof
- sense of providence, or the lack thereof
- faith, or the lack thereof
- a sense of grace or gratefulness, in contrast to a lack of appreciation and entitlement
- repentance, versus unrepentant stance toward others and the world
- communion (or feeling part of a whole), or on the continuum toward sensing no connection with others or the world
- sense of vocation (purpose) versus meaninglessness.

Although this model is clearly influenced by a Christian worldview and may therefore be limited in its applicability, it offers a good approach to thinking about spirituality comprehensively.

Standardized Questionnaires

Paper-and-pencil–type questionnaires for measuring spirituality for research abound; some also have been recommended for clinical assessment purposes. This approach to conducting a spiritual assessment allows for identification, and possibly measurement, of how one spiritually believes, belongs, and behaves. This type of tool, however, should not "stand alone" in the spiritual assessment process; rather, it can be the springboard for a more thorough patient assessment and deeper encounter, as appropriate. A quantitative tool should never replace human contact, but instead should facilitate it. Although a quantitative spiritual self-assessment form provides an opportunity for healthcare teams to glean substantial spiritual belief/practice information, it is limited by its mechanistic, rigid, and non-individualized nature.

For example, the Functional Assessment of Chronic Illness Therapy-Spiritual Well-being (FACIT-Sp) is a short 12-item instrument that assesses both religious and existential/spiritual well-being. Example items include "I feel peaceful" and "I am able to reach down deep into myself for comfort." The 5-point response options range from "not at all" to "very much." It has been used extensively for health-related research purposes.[33] More recent testing suggests the tool measures not only faith (religious well-being) and meaning (existential/spiritual well-being), but also peace.[34] The FACIT-Sp has received considerable validation in numerous studies among persons with cancer.

The Daily Spiritual Experience (DSE) Scale is another possible standardized screening tool.[35] Designed to measure "the individual's perception of the transcendent (God, the divine) in daily life and the perception of interaction with, or involvement of, the transcendent in life rather than particular beliefs or behaviors, [it is] intended to transcend the boundaries of any particular religion" (p. 23). The DSE is a 16-item scale with Likert-type response options measuring frequency. Like the FACIT-Sp, this research instrument has been used often in investigating patient spiritual responses and has well-established validity.

More recently developed for patients in general is the Spiritual Needs Assessment for Patients (SNAP).[36] This tool was likewise systematically developed, psychometrically tested, and found to have good support for its validity and reliability. It comprises 5 items assessing a psychosocial domain (e.g., needs related to "sharing your thoughts and feelings with people close to you"), 13 items measuring spirituality (e.g., needs related to "resolving old disputes, hurts or resentments among family and friends"), and 5 items about religious needs (e.g., "religious rituals such as chant, prayer, lighting candles or incense, anointing, or communion"). Response options range from "1" (not at all) to "4" (very much).

The Brief RCOPE, developed by Pargament and colleagues, is a 14-item instrument that measures the degree of positive and negative religious coping.[37] This tool evolved from a longer version and a program of research examining the psychology of religious coping. Substantial psychometric testing affirms the validity of the tool. Positive religious coping subscale items refer to a secure attachment to God, a sense of connectedness, and benevolence. The negative religious coping subscale items inquire about abandonment and punishment by God, isolation from faith community, the power of God, and attributing poor coping to the Devil. Pargament's program of research firmly establishes negative religious coping as maladaptive, and positive religious coping as adaptive, in illness contexts.

Although not so brief, the Royal Free Interview Schedule developed in the United Kingdom by King, Speck, and Thomas[38] is a 2½-page self-report questionnaire. The tool showed acceptable reliability and various forms of validity, when it was tested among 297 persons who were primarily hospital employees and church members. Questionnaire items assess both spiritual and religious "understanding in life" (1 item), religious/spiritual beliefs (8 items), religious/spiritual practices (3 items), and "intense" spiritual or "near death" experiences (6 items). Response options for items include Likert scales, categorical options, and space for answering open-ended questions.

Whereas these tools may offer the best approaches to a quantification of spiritual needs in a palliative care setting, other tools do exist. For further discussion of these tools (mostly developed for research purposes), see the reviews provided by Monod and colleagues,[39] Draper,[40] and Lunder and colleagues.[41] Monod and colleagues observed that only 2 of the 35 scales measuring the spiritual could have clinical usefulness. If spirituality is indeed a vital sign, as Lunder and colleagues posit, then careful consideration should be given to how nurses can screen and assess this vital essence of personhood.

Other Spiritual Assessment Methods

Other approaches to spiritual assessment have been described in addition to the interview and questionnaire techniques. LeFavi and Wessels[42] described how life reviews can become, in essence, spiritual assessments. Life reviews are especially valuable for persons who are dying, as they allow patients to make sense of and reconcile their life story. By doing a life review with a terminally ill patient, the nurse can assess many dimensions of spirituality (e.g., worldviews, commitments, missions, values) in a natural, noncontrived manner. Life reviews can be prompted by questions about the significant events, people, and challenges during the life span. A life review can also occur when inquiring about personal objects, pictures, or other memorabilia the patient wants to share.

Chochinov and various colleagues around the world have developed and tested Dignity Therapy, which allows persons at the end of life an opportunity to do a life review.[43] The semistructured questions of Dignity Therapy include: "Tell me a little about your life history, particularly the parts you either remember most or think are most important? When did you feel most alive? Are there specific things that you would want your family to know about you . . . ? What are the most important roles you have played in life . . . ? What are your most important accomplishments . . . ? Are there particular things that you feel still need to be said . . . ? What are your hopes and dreams for your loved ones? What have you learned about life that you would want to pass along . . . ? Are there other things that you would like included?" The patient response to these questions, asked by a trained volunteer, are recorded and transcribed into a permanent record that the patient helps design and can leave as a legacy for loved ones. Although Dignity Therapy is reminiscence therapy, these questions overlap with those asked in a comprehensive spiritual assessment.

Hodge[21] identified several creative approaches to collecting information about client spirituality. As a social worker, Hodge is well aware that some patients are not verbal or comfortable expressing their spirituality in words. He explained more visual ways for a patient to describe his or her spiritual experiences. Such methods include:

- Spiritual lifemaps or a pictorial depiction of where the patient has been spiritually, is presently, and expects to go. It can be a simple pencil drawing on a large piece of paper; words and illustrations can be used to convey the spiritual story—the spiritual highs and lows, blessings and burdens.

- Spiritual genograms, like a standard genogram, depict the issues and influences over one to three generations. Sources of spiritual influence from certain relationships (including those external to the family) can be drawn. Words that identify key spiritual beliefs and practices transmitted via relationships, and significant spiritual events that contribute to the patient's spiritual life, can be noted around this spiritual family tree.

- Spiritual ecomaps, rather than focusing on past spiritual influences, direct the patient to consider present spiritual experiences. In particular, the patient can diagram (with himself or herself portrayed in the center) the relationship with God or a transcendent other/value, rituals, faith community, and encounters with other spiritual entities.

- Spiritual ecograms allow the patient to diagram present perspectives on both family and spiritual relationships; it is a fusion of the spiritual genogram and ecomap.[40]

- Other strategies include having clients draw a spiritual timeline that includes significant books, experiences, and events. Another unusual approach involves sentence completion. For example, a client may fill in the blank of sentences like "My relation to God . . ." or "What I would really like to be . . ." or "When I feel overwhelmed. . . ." Having verbally oriented assessment strategies as well as nonverbal methods provides clinicians with a toolbox for assessing spirituality, allowing the clinician to choose an approach that fits the patient's personality, circumstances, and purpose for assessment.

Summary of Spiritual Screening and Assessment Models

Box 1.3 provides a case study to illustrate a few spiritual screening approaches. Comparing the four screening techniques reveals that different data were generated from each. It should be remembered that each approach to spiritual assessment is one lens and may not address other important areas of spirituality (e.g., spiritually comforting practices and preparation for death are omitted from the FICA and MVAST approaches).

The models in Box 1.3 identify spiritual dimensions that may be included in a spiritual assessment. Many of the dimensions identified in one model are observed (often using different language) in other models. Except for Hodge's[40] diagrammatic methods, these assessment approaches generally require the professional to make observations while asking questions and listening to the patient's response. The vast majority of recommended questions are open-ended. Several of the questions—indeed, the dimensions of spirituality—identified in this literature use "God language" or assume a patient will believe in some transcendent divinity. These models are developed by professionals who are influenced predominantly by Western, Judeo-Christian ways of thinking.

Box 1.3 Case Study: Mr. T, Entering Hospice Service with Parkinson's Disease

History

Mr. T is a 74-year-old Protestant gentleman who was diagnosed about 13 years ago with Parkinson's disease. Until 8 months ago, he lived alone. When he realized he could no longer safely live alone, he moved to an assisted living facility. Now his condition has deteriorated further, requiring his admission to a skilled nursing facility. This facility has obtained hospice services for Mr. T. He is receiving anti-parkinsonian and anti-depressive medications.

Mr. T is divorced from his third wife and estranged from his only son and a stepson. The son lives 7 hours away (by car), and usually reenters Mr. T's life when he needs financial assistance. The only family that appears to show interest in supporting Mr. T is a niece and her husband, who live 2 hours away. Since Mr. T's divorce 10 years ago, he has been befriended by a middle-aged woman, Darlene, who has entered several business ventures with Mr. T's money.

The following are excerpts from conversations the author had with Mr. T:

"My dad was a doctor. He practiced until he was 91! He was very respected and well-known. He loved to yacht; he won the Trans-Pac race one year. I was a teen then, and could only travel with him if I was the crew's cook. So my mom taught me to peel potatoes . . . !

"I wanted to be a doctor. I just couldn't get the grades, got kicked out of college . . . never could have gotten into med school. So I sold cookware instead. But they said I could sell snow in Alaska—I was good at selling. . . .

(continued)

Box 1.3 (Continued)

CHAPTER 1 **Spiritual Assessment**

15

"I was born and raised in the church. Went to Christian schools all the way through college. I was an elder at my little church before I moved down here. I've got the church even in my will. . . .

"I know Darlene is using me, but I love her. I would marry her if I could. [She was married.] My head says one thing, but my heart says another. . . .

"I remember once making love to a woman and her reaction was, 'Oh my God!' I guess that was a spiritual experience I helped her have!

"There's not much for me to do here. Just a bunch of old people around here. Sometimes I wonder, 'Why? Why keep going?' . . . I don't have anymore money to give. . . . My body doesn't work anymore. . . .

[During a phone call when Mr. T related he felt anxious:] "I'm having a hard time . . . really worried about how it's all going to end. How will it? . . . [When asked, "How at peace do you feel inside?":] Not at all. [When asked, "Is there anything you can think of that would bring comfort to you now?":] No, nothing."

Screening (using FICA)

- F (faith)—verbalized about some indicators of adherence to a faith tradition; inward (or intrinsic) faith is fundamentally challenged as he faces his end; his faith appears to lean toward an extrinsic faith (e.g., attendance at services, donating money).
- I (importance)—states it is important.
- C (community)—until institutionalized, was a leader in a local Seventh-day Adventist congregation; desires to continue to attend.
- A (address)—readily responds positively to query regarding having local pastor visit him; also accepts offer of loaned spiritual viewing materials (e.g., videos of dramatized Gospels) and musical CDs. When asked how the staff can spiritually support, he states, "No, they don't need to butt into this part of my life."

Screening (using MVAST)

- Moral authority—He states the Bible is the guide for what is right or wrong. He admits struggling about how to morally relate to Darlene and yearns to reconnect with his sons.
- Vocational—He excelled as a salesman during mid-adult years. More recently, his business ventures have failed. During his youth, he aspired to be a physician, yet failed to attain that goal. His life seems to have been lived in the shadow of his father's, perhaps challenging his sense of worth. His financial failure also seems to challenge his sense of success and purposefulness.
- Aesthetic—Loves "cars, motorcycles, and beautiful women!" His disease now prevents his ability to enjoy these interests, as he can no longer drive or attract women for a date. He does enjoy eating and listening to jazz.

(continued)

Box 1.3 (Continued)

- Social—until institutionalized, was a leader in a local Seventh-day Adventist congregation; desires to continue to attend as he enjoys the opportunity to see old friends and meet people there.

- Transcendent—says he prays before each meal and at bedtime, and then at times when he is very distressed, but reports that "sometimes it feels like the prayers don't go anywhere." Never describes a time in his life when there was an affective experience of God; rather, his descriptions of religious experience seem cerebral and proscribed. He does describe several times in his life when he believes his life was spared, and interprets these events as showing God intervening in his life.

Screening using FACIT-Sp:

Mr. T's score might indicate low peace, low existential/spiritual well-being, and perhaps slightly higher (but still low) religious well-being.

Screening using Brief RCOPE:

Mr. T's score likely would have indicated moderately high negative religious coping and low positive religious coping.

Reproduced by permission of Oxford University Press USA from Taylor EJ. Spiritual assessment. In: Ferrell BR, Coyle N, eds. *Oxford Textbook of Palliative Nursing.* 4th ed., New York, NY: Oxford University Press; 2015:539 (Box 32.2).

General Observations and Suggestions for Conducting a Spiritual Assessment

When to Assess

The spiritual assessment consensus project advocated that spiritual screening be done at admission and whenever the patient's status changed.[16] Furthermore, when the spiritual screening suggests potential for spiritual distress, a trained chaplain should be called within 24 hours for a more complete assessment. Spiritual assessment should be an ongoing process. The nurse does not complete a spiritual assessment simply by asking questions about religion or spirituality during an intake interview. Rather, spiritual assessment should continue throughout the nurse–patient relationship. A nurse trained in how spiritual health is manifested will be able to see and hear patient spirituality, as it is embedded in and suffuses the everyday encounter.[44]

Gaining Entrée

Spiritual needs are complex and often difficult to acknowledge, and more so to describe in words. The patient may not feel comfortable divulging such inner, heart-touching experience and intimate information to a nurse with whom rapport has not been established.

Two studies provide evidence regarding what patients are looking for in a clinician, if they are going to talk openly about their spirituality.[45,46] Survey responses from cancer patients and family caregivers (N = 224) about what requisites they would want in a nurse who provided spiritual care revealed that relationship (i.e., "show me kindness and respect" and "get to know me first") was ranked highest, with a nurse's training in spiritual care or sharing similar beliefs as less important.[47] Likewise, a small qualitative study of chronically and terminally ill patients observed that these respondents viewed relational characteristics (e.g., caring, honor and respect, rapport/ trust) as prerequisites for discussing spirituality with a physician.[46] Ellis's and Campbell's study identified other factors that patients perceive facilitate physician spiritual assessment: a conducive setting, sharing of the patient's life priorities or values, perceived physician receptivity to spiritual questions, and sensing that the physician considered spiritual health to be integral to health.[48]

Because spirituality and religiosity are sensitive and personal topics (as are most other topics nurses assess), it is polite for a nurse to preface a spiritual assessment with an acknowledgment of the sensitivity of the questions and an explanation of why an assessment is necessary.[44,49] For example, Maugens[49] suggested this preface: Many people have strong spiritual or religious beliefs that shape their lives, including their health and experiences with illness. If you are comfortable talking about this topic, would you please share any of your beliefs and practices that you might want me to know as your physician (p. 12)? Undoubtedly, such a preface will help both the patient and the clinician feel at ease during the assessment.

Assessing Nonverbal Indicators of Spirituality

Although this spiritual assessment discussion has thus far focused on how to frame a verbal question and allow a patient to verbalize a response, the nurse must remember that most communication occurs nonverbally and the nurse must assess this nonverbal communication and the environment of the patient as well.[2,3,44] Does the patient appear agitated or angry? What does body language convey? What is the speed and tone of voice? Assessment of the patient's environment can provide clues about spiritual state. Are there religious objects on the bedside table? Are there religious paintings or crucifixes on the walls? Are there get-well cards or books with spiritual themes? Are there indicators that the patient has many friends and family providing love and a sense of community? Are the curtains closed and the bedspread pulled over the face? Many of the factors a palliative care nurse assesses as a matter of course will provide spiritual assessment data, in addition to the psychosocial assessment.

Language: Religious or Spiritual Words?

One barrier to spiritual assessment is the nurse's fear of offending a nonreligious patient by using religious language. However, when one remembers the nonreligious nature of spirituality, this barrier disappears. Patient spirituality can be discussed without reference to God and religion. Also, using the terms *need* or *distress* immediately after *spiritual* could be denigrating for a patient. Especially with spirituality, patients may be upset when they hear others consider them needy.

Nurses can easily avoid offensive jargon. First, the nurse can begin the assessment with general questions, unrelated to religious assumptions. For example, "What is giving you the strength to cope with your illness now?" or "What spiritual beliefs and practices are important to you, as you cope with your illness?" Second, the nurse must listen for the language of the patient and use it to formulate more specific follow-up questions. If a patient responds to a question with "My faith and prayers help me," then the nurse knows *faith* and *prayer* are words that will not offend this patient. If a patient states that the "Great Spirit guides," then the sensitive nurse will not respond with, "Tell me how Jesus is your guide." Questions using nonreligious language are presented in Box 1.4.

Asking Questions

Because questioning a patient is integral in most spiritual assessments, it is good to remember the basics of formulating good questions. When a nurse has no time or ability to assess further, he or she may find that asking closed-ended questions provides short factual or yes/no responses. Otherwise, to appreciate the uniqueness and complexity of an individual's spirituality, the nurse must ask open-ended questions. The best questions begin with *how, what, when, who*, or phrases like "Tell me about. . . ." Generally, questions beginning with *why* are not helpful; they often threaten or challenge (e.g., "Why do you believe that?").[44]

Box 1.4 A Collection of Nonreligious Questions to Broach the Topic of Spirituality With Palliative Care Patients

You've gone through so much lately. Where do you get your inner strength and courage to keep going?

What is helping you to cope?

What comforts are most satisfying for you now?

As you think about your future, what worries you most?

Some people seem more to live while they are dying, while others seem to die while they are living. Which way is it for you? What makes it that way?

What kind of person do you see yourself as? (Note: Chaplains suggest that how one views self parallels how one views their Creator or God.)

What do you see as the purpose for your life now, given your body isn't allowing you to do all you used to do?

What hopes and dreams do you have for your future? For your family?

What legacy would you like to leave? How can we make sure that that happens?

As I've gotten to know you, I've noticed you speak often of (spiritual theme [e.g., betrayal, yearning for love]). How do you think this theme has influenced your life, or will influence your future? How happy with your life's theme are you?

Tell me about times during your life where you faced a huge challenge. What got you through? Is that resource still available to you now?

Reprinted by permission of SAGE Publications from Dudley JR, Smith C, Millison MB. Unfinished business: Assessing the spiritual needs of hospice clients. *Am J Hospice Palliat Care.* 1995;12:30–37.

Listening to the Answers

The palliative care nurse must remember the importance of listening to the patient's responses. Remember that silence has an appropriate role when listening to a patient's spiritual and sacred story.[44] Remain neutral, nonjudgmental. View the patient as a fellow sojourner on the journey of life. Recognize that you are not the authority or savior for the patient expressing spiritual pain. Rather, you are a companion or a supporter, if so privileged. Listen for more than words; metaphors, a spiritual theme that keeps reemerging throughout life stories. Listen to where the patient places energy and for emotion in addition to cognitions. The nurse will do well to listen to his or her own inner response, which will mirror the feelings of the patient.[44]

Overcoming the Time Barrier

Healthcare professionals may believe that they do not have enough time to conduct a spiritual assessment. Indeed, Maugens[49] observed that completing a patient's spiritual history took about 10 to 15 minutes. Although this is much less time than Maugens and his colleagues expected, it is still a considerable amount of time in today's healthcare context. One response to this time barrier is to remember that spiritual assessment is a process that develops, as the nurse gains the patient's trust. The nurse can accomplish the assessment during "clinical chatterings."[49] Furthermore, data for a spiritual assessment can be collected simultaneously with other assessments or during interventions (e.g., while bathing or completing bedtime care). And finally, it can be argued that nurses do not have time not to conduct a spiritual assessment, considering the fundamental and powerful nature of spirituality. Skalla and McCoy (a nurse and a chaplain) remind the users of their MVAST model that the questions are a guide, and not prescriptive; they can be threaded into the natural course of a conversation.[50]

Overcoming Personal Barriers

Nurses can encounter their own personal barriers in conducting a spiritual assessment. These barriers may include feelings of embarrassment or insecurity about the topic or can result from projection of unresolved and painful personal spiritual doubts or struggles. Every nurse has a personal philosophy or worldview that influences his or her spiritual beliefs. These beliefs can color or blind the nurse's assessment techniques and interpretation. Hence, an accurate and sensitive spiritual assessment presumably correlates with the degree of the nurse's spiritual self-awareness. Put another way, one's ability to hear one's own spiritual story is directly related to one's ability to hear a patient's spiritual story.[44] Nurses can increase their comfort with the topic and their awareness of their spiritual self by asking themselves variations of the questions they anticipate asking patients. For example, "What gives my life meaning and purpose?" "How do my spiritual beliefs influence the way I relate to my own death?" "How do I love myself and forgive myself?" Recognizing how one's spiritual beliefs motivate one's vocation as a nurse is also extremely helpful.

Concluding Cautions

Although the models and evidence supporting spiritual assessment imply that it is a non-problematic and simple process, it would be naive to leave this impression. Several experts suggest potential problems associated with spiritual assessment. These include:

- The process of taking spiritual assessment data to make a spiritual diagnosis pathologizes what may be a normal process of spiritual growth.[51] Assessment tools often assume that spiritual well-being correlates with feeling good; spiritual health and suffering cannot coexist.[6] (A more appropriate way to evaluate spirituality may be to ask how harmful one's spirituality is to self and others.[44])

- A "tick box" approach to spiritual assessment could freeze patient spirituality at the time when the assessment was completed; spiritual assessment would be considered complete and not continue.[51]

- A fairly prescribed assessment tool could disempower a patient. That is, the clinician controls (overpowers) the agenda by determining what spiritual matters are discussed.[52] An assessment tool could limit and control patient expression.[53]

- A spiritual assessment to some degree will reflect the assumptions influencing the clinician (a major one being that spirituality is universal). Thus, a spiritual worldview may be imposed on a vulnerable patient. An ethical spiritual assessment would be nonalienating, nondiscriminating, and engage and respect the patient.[54,55] Indeed, existent standardized spiritual assessment tools generally have not been tested in many cultures, so it is unknown how culturally appropriate or sensitive they are.[41]

Thus, a spiritual assessment tool—if a tool is needed—should be able to generate helpful data for guiding patient care, encourage patient participation, be flexible and easy to use, take little clinician time, be nonintrusive, allow for a patient's unique story to be understood to some degree, and be simple and clear.[55] A tall ask? Perhaps. But important to strive toward.

Assessing Special Populations

Assessing Impaired Patients

Although verbal conversation is integral to a typical spiritual assessment, some terminally ill patients may not be able to speak, hear, or understand a verbal assessment. Patients who are unable to communicate verbally may feel unheard. In such situations, the nurse must remember alternative sources of information. She or he can consult with the family members and observe the patient's environment and nonverbal communications. For example, Telos[56] proposed that for some patients, terminal restlessness was a manifestation of spiritual distress. Ruling out other causes, and relying on previous spiritual assessment opportunities that have revealed unresolved spiritual issues, supports this conclusion. (Hence, the importance of proactively conducting spiritual assessments for those with terminal illness.) Alternative methods for "conversing" can also be used. For patients who can write, paper-and-pencil questionnaires can be very helpful. Always be patient and unafraid of the tears that can follow. Questions that demonstrate concern for patients' innermost well-being may release their floodgates for tears.

For persons with dementia or other cognitive impairments, it is helpful to recognize that communication can still occur on an emotional or physical level if not intellectually. Their disjointed stories will still offer you a window into their world. Even if you cannot sew the pieces together, trying will help you remain curious and engaged.[44]

Assessing Children

Several strategies can be employed to assess a child's spirituality. The clinician must remember, however, that building trust and rapport with children is essential to completing a helpful spiritual assessment. Children are especially capable of ascertaining an adult's degree of authenticity and less likely to be offended by a question about religion. If a nurse creates a comfortable and nonjudgmental atmosphere in which a child can discuss spiritual topics, then the child will talk. Never underestimate the profoundness of a child's spiritual experience, especially a dying child's.

In addition to asking questions verbally, the nurse can use play interviews, picture drawings, observations, and informal interviews.[57] The nurse may need to be more creative in formulating questions if the child's vocabulary is limited. For example, instead of asking the child about helpful religious rituals, the nurse can ask questions about what they do to get ready to sleep or what they do on weekends. When asking, "Does your mommy pray with you before you go to sleep?" or "What do you do on Sunday or Sabbath mornings?" the nurse can learn whether prayer or religious service attendance are a part of this child's life. An assessment question that Sexson's[57] colleague, Patricia Fosarelli, found to be particularly helpful with 6- to 18-year-olds was: "If you could get God to answer one question, what one question would you ask God?"

While assessing children, it is vital to consider their stage of cognitive and faith development.[57,58] Questions must be framed in age-appropriate language (a 4-year-old will likely not understand what "spiritual belief" means!). Toddlers and preschoolers talk about their spirituality in very concrete terms, in an egocentric manner. School-age and adolescent children should be addressed straightforwardly about how they see their illness. Inquiring about the cause of their illness is especially important, as many children view their illness and impending death as punishment.

As with adults, children's nonverbal behaviors provide significant information in a spiritual screening or assessment. Mueller[58] advises that extensive crying, withdrawal, and regressive and resistant behaviors are potential indicators of spiritual distress. Likewise, difficulty eating or sleeping (nightmares) and somatic complaints can reflect spiritual distress.

Assessing Families

Understanding the family's spirituality is pivotal to understanding the child's. Structured interviews or unstructured conversations with parents and even older siblings will inform the healthcare team about the child's spirituality.[57,59] Similarly, knowing the spiritual or religious family context of an adult patient can also inform clinicians about a patient's faith context. Studies document that the spiritual distress of family caregivers is not unlike that of their beloved.[12,60,61] Given the provision of 24/7 physical care, the unrelenting uncertainty and anxiety, and the constellation of stressors family caregivers endure, it is not surprising they may feel angry at God,[12] isolated from their faith community, and challenged to have a meaningful outlook on life.[60] Indeed, in Delgado Guay and colleagues' study, 58% of family caregivers surveyed reported some spiritual pain.[61] Although it is highly unlikely that a nurse will be completing a comprehensive spiritual assessment of a family, an awareness of this process can give the nurse a richer perspective with which to conduct a screening, when it is appropriate.

Barnes and colleagues[62] suggested the following questions as guides for assessing how a family's spirituality affects illness experience:

- How does the family understand life's purpose and meaning?
- How do they explain illness and suffering?
- How do they view the person in the context of the body, mind, soul, spirit?
- How is the specific illness of the child explained?
- What treatments are necessary for the child?
- Who is the qualified person to address these various treatments for the child's healing?
- What is the outcome measurement that the family is using to measure successful treatment (good death)?

Ferrell and Baird[63] offer several family spiritual assessment questions that are specific to the caregiving role many family members perform:

- We recognize that often family caregivers' spirituality may be similar to or very different from the patient's spirituality. Are there spiritual needs you have as a family caregiver?
- Many family caregivers tell us that while caring for a loved one is very difficult, caregiving can also be a very meaningful experience. What has it been like for you? (p. 257)

These questions will likely be welcomed by the family caregiver who is engaged in providing health-related care to a loved one. Asking such questions will acknowledge to this caregiver that his or her role is recognized and appreciated. It will also provide the family caregiver opportunity to express and reflect on his or her own needs.

Buck and McMillan took the Spiritual Needs Inventory (SNI) developed by Hermann for patients, and tested its validity with 410 family caregivers of hospice patients.[60] This 17-item instrument assesses religious needs (e.g., for devotional practices and service attendance), outlook needs (e.g., "think happy thoughts," "be with friends," "see smiles"), and community needs (e.g., knowing about or being with family and friends). The SNI offers a possible method for a standardized approach to family caregiver spiritual screening and assessment.

Assessing Diverse Spiritualities

Spiritual assessment methods must be flexible enough for use with persons of diverse spiritual and religious backgrounds. Although the questions and assumptions presented in this chapter will be helpful for assessing most patients living in Western, Euro-American cultures, they may not be helpful for patients who do not share these presuppositions. For example, some may believe it is wrong to discuss their inner spiritual turmoil as they face death and will refuse to fully engage in the spiritual assessment process. (Whereas some Buddhists and Hindus may believe they must be in a peaceful state to be reincarnated to a better state, African American Christians may think it is sinful to express doubts or anger toward God.) Framing spiritual assessment in a positive tone may overcome this type of barrier (e.g., "Tell me about how you are at peace now.") Others may assume they are void of spirituality and therefore decline any questions regarding their "spirituality." This barrier to assessment can be overcome with questions that omit such language (e.g., "What gives your life meaning?" or "How is your courage?").

For patients who are religious, it is important to remember that no two members of a religious community are exactly alike.[3] Although a cursory understanding of the world's major religious traditions provides nurses with some framework for inquiry, remaining open to the variation of religious experience and expression is essential.

The Next Step: What to Do With a Spiritual Assessment

Interpreting the Data

A spiritual screening can generate a lot of information. This information must be processed to identify what, if any, spiritual need exists and then to plan spiritual care. Several points can be considered while processing the data. These include:

- What patients tell you at first reflects not how well you have asked a good question; rather, it shows how safe and respected the patient feels with you.

- Consider what incongruities exist. Do the affect, behavior, and communication (ABCs) line up?

- Consider the level of concreteness or abstractness in the patient's talk about spiritual matters. Healthy spirituality resides between these opposites.

- Consider how defensive or threatened the patient is by discussing spirituality. Did the patient change the topic? Give superficial answers? Become competitive? Intellectualize feelings?

- Keep in mind that crises (e.g., illness) expose gaps in a patient's spiritual development. Did significant events earlier in life stunt the patient's spiritual growth?

- Remember that religion offers a lens for interpreting life. Likewise, when patients tell meaningful stories, legends, or passages from their holy scripture, they are telling you about themselves.
- Reflect on how helpful versus harmful a patient's spiritual beliefs and practices are. Do they create inner anxiety? Do they limit the patient from using other helpful coping strategies? [44]

Although an in-depth analysis is beyond the scope of most palliative care nurses, having an awareness of the ways to evaluate what a patient says will help the nurse begin to make sense of the data.

Documentation

Although assessments of physiological phenomena are readily documented in patient charts, assessments and diagnoses of spiritual problems are less frequently documented. For many reasons, however, spiritual assessments and care should be documented. These reasons include (1) facilitating the continuity of patient care among palliative care team members and (2) documenting for the monitoring purposes of accrediting bodies, researchers, and quality improvement teams. Power[51] recognized that the data collected during spiritual assessments is often very private, sensitive material; to document such may breach confidentiality and thus pose an ethical dilemma. As with other sensitive charted information, nurses must treat spiritual assessment data with respect and observe applicable privacy codes.

Formats for documenting spiritual assessments and diagnoses vary. Some institutions encourage staff to use SOAP (Subjective, Objective, Assessment, Plan) or similar formatting in progress notes shared by the multidisciplinary team. Others have developed quick and easy checklists for documenting spiritual and religious issues. Perhaps an assessment format that allows for both rapid documentation and optional narrative data is best. However, merely documenting one's religious affiliation and desire for a referral to a spiritual care specialist does not adequately indicate a patient's spiritual status and need.

Institutional Approaches to Spiritual Screening and Assessment

A 2-year demonstration project to improve spiritual assessment in palliative care settings was recently completed.[64,65] Funded by the Archstone Foundation and convened by the City of Hope National Medical Center, this project provided significant funding to nine southern California healthcare organizations with palliative care services. This project allowed experts to share information, resources, and change strategies with each site, so they could better institute spiritual assessment and spiritual care.

Each site, of course, developed its unique method, constructing a screening tool that comprised a very few open-ended screening questions. These questions were embedded into the healthcare system's standardized admission assessment, usually electronically. The electronic medical record system was designed to allow the clinician not only to insert patient responses to screening questions (sometimes requiring the nurse to translate a qualitative response into a yes/no tick box response), but also to submit a referral or add to a care plan, if a spiritual need was identified. Palliative care service clinicians were educated at each site about spiritual screening, the newly implemented process for screening, and how to document patient spiritual status.[66]

Chapter Summary

Spirituality is an elemental and pervading dimension, especially for those whose death is imminent. Spiritual assessment is essential to effective and sensitive spiritual care, and indeed is the beginning of spiritual care. While the nurse questions a patient about spirituality, she or he simultaneously assists the patient in reflecting on the innermost and most important aspects of being human, while indicating to the patient that grappling with spiritual issues is normal and valuable. During this assessment, the nurse is providing spiritual care by being present and witnessing what is sacred for the patient.

References

1. Reed PG. An emerging paradigm for the investigation of spirituality in nursing. *Res Nurs Health.* 1992;15:349–357.

2. Puchalski CM, Ferrell B. *Making Health Care Whole: Integrating Spirituality Into Patient Care.* West Conshohocken, PA: Templeton Press; 2010.

3. Taylor EJ. *Religion: A Clinical Guide for Nurses.* New York: Springer; 2012.

4. Narayansamy A. The puzzle of spirituality for nursing: a guide to practical assessment. *Br J Nurs.* 2004;13(19):1140–1144.

5. Paley J. Spirituality and secularization: nursing and the sociology of religion. *J Clin Nurs.* 2008;17:175–186.

6. Pesut B, Fowler M, Reimer-Kirkham S, Taylor EJ, Sawatzky R. Particularizing spirituality in points of tension. *Nurs Inquiry.* 2009;16:337–346.

7. Bash A. Spirituality: the emperor's new clothes? *J Clin Nurs.* 2004;13:11–16.

8. McSherry W, Ross L. Dilemmas of spiritual assessment: considerations for nursing practice. *J Adv Nurs.* 2002;38:479–488.

9. Williams AL. Perspectives on spirituality at the end of life: A meta-summary. *Palliat Support Care.* 2006;4:407–417.

10. Taylor EJ. Spiritual responses to cancer. In: Yarbro CH, Wujcik D, Gobel BH, eds. *Cancer Nursing: Principles and Practice.* 7th ed. Sudbury, MA: Jones & Bartlett; 2010:1797–1812.

11. Taylor EJ, Davenport F. Spiritual quality of life. In: King CR, Hinds PS, eds. *Quality of Life: From Nursing and Patient Perspectives.* 3rd ed. Sudbury, MA: Jones & Bartlett; 2012:83–104.

12. Exline JJ, Prince-Paul M, Root BL, Peereboom KS. The spiritual struggle of anger toward God: a study with family members of hospice patients. *J Palliat Med.* 2013;16:369–375.

13. Newberry AG, Choi CW, Donovan HS, et al. Exploring spirituality in family caregivers of patients with primary malignant brain tumors across the disease trajectory. *Oncol Nurs Forum*. 2013;40(3):E119–E125.

14. National Consensus Project for Quality Palliative Care. *Clinical Practice Guidelines for Quality Palliative Care*. 3rd ed. Pittsburgh, PA: National Consensus Project for Quality Palliative Care; 2013. http://www.nationalconsensusproject.org. Accessed July 2, 2013.

15. The Joint Commission. Spiritual assessment. Joint Commission Web site. http://www.jointcommission.org/mobile. Accessed December 31, 2008.

16. Puchalski C, Ferrell B, Virani R, et al. Improving the quality of spiritual care as a dimension of palliative care: the report of the Consensus Conference. *J Palliat Med*. 2009;12(10):885–904.

17. Kalish N. Evidence-based spiritual care: A literature review. *Curr Opin Support Palliat Care*. 2012;6:242–246.

18. Taylor EJ. New Zealand hospice nurses' self-rated comfort in conducting spiritual assessment. *Int J Palliat Care Nurs*. 2013;19:178–185.

19. Cobb M, Dowrick C, Lloyd-Williams M. What can we learn about the spiritual needs of palliative care patients from the research literature? *J Pain Symp Manag*. 2012;43:1105–1119.

20. Hodge DR. Administering a two-stage spiritual assessment in healthcare settings: a necessary component of ethical and effective care. *J Nurs Manag*. 2013; 21(3):403–404.

21. Hodge D. Developing a spiritual assessment toolbox: A discussion of the strengths and limitations of five different assessment methods. *Health Soc Work*. 2005;10:314–323.

22. Kub JE, Nolan MT, Hughes MT, et al. Religious importance and practices of patients with a life-threatening illness: implications for screening protocols. *Appl Nurs Res*. 2003;16:196–200.

23. Lawrence RT, Smith DW. Principles to make a spiritual assessment work in your practice. *J Fam Pract*. 2004;53:625–631.

24. Steinhauser KE, Voils CI, Clipp EC, Bosworth HB, Christakis NA, Tulsky JA. "Are you at peace?": One item to probe spiritual concerns at the end of life. *Arch Intern Med* 2006;166(1):101–105.

25. Lo B, Quill T, Tulsky J. Discussing palliative care with patients. *Ann Intern Med*. 1999;130:744–749.

26. Matthews DA, McCullough ME, Larson DB, Koenig HG, Swyers JP, Milano MG. Religious commitment and health status: a review of the research and implications for family medicine. *Arch Fam Med*. 1998;7:118–124.

27. Borneman T, Ferrell B, Puchalski CM. Evaluation of the FICA Tool for Spiritual Assessment. *J Pain Symp Manag*. 2010;40:163–173.

28. Hodge D. A template for spiritual assessment: a review of the JCAHO requirements and guidelines for implementation. *Soc Work*. 2006;51:317–326.

29. Frick E, Riedner C, Fegg MJ, Hauf S, Borasio GD. A clinical interview assessing cancer patients' spiritual needs and preferences. *Eur J Cancer Care (Engl)*. 2006;15:238–243.

30. Taylor EJ. Religion and patient care. In: Fowler M, Kirkham-Reimer S, Sawatzky R, Taylor EJ, eds. *Religion, Religious Ethics, and Nursing*. New York, NY: Springer; 2011:313–338.

31. Fitchett G. *Assessing Spiritual Needs: A Guide for Caregivers*. Lima, OH: Academic Renewal Press; 2002.

32. Pruyser, P. *The Minister as Diagnostician: Personal Problems in Pastoral Perspective*. Philadelphia, PA: Westminster Press; 1976.

33. Peterman A, Fitchett G, Brady MJ, Hernandez L, Cella D. Measuring spiritual well-being in people with cancer: The Functional Assessment of Chronic Illness Therapy-Spiritual Well-Being Scale (FACIT-Sp). *Ann Behav Med*. 2002;24(1):49–58.

34. Murphy PE, Canada AL, Fitchett G, et al. An examination of the 3-factor model and structural invariance across racial/ethnic groups for the FACIT-Sp: a report from the American Cancer Society's Study of Cancer Survivors-II (SCS-II). *Psychooncol*. 2010;19:264–272.

35. Underwood LG, Teresi JA. The Daily Spiritual Experience Scale: Development, theoretical description, reliability, exploratory factor analysis, and preliminary construct validity using health-related data. *Ann Behav Med*. 2002;24(1):22–33.

36. Sharma RK, Astrow AB, Texeira K, Sulmasy DP. The Spiritual Needs Assessment for Patients (SNAP): development and validation of a comprehensive instrument to assess unmet spiritual needs. *J Pain Symp Manag*. 2012;44:44–51.

37. Pargament K, Feuille M, Burdzy D. The Brief RCOPE: Current psychometric status of a short measure of religious coping. *Religions*. 2011;2(1):51–76.

38. King M, Speck P, Thomas A. The Royal Free Interview for spiritual and religious beliefs: development and validation of a self-report version. *Psychol Med*. 2001;31:1015–1023.

39. Monod S, Brennan M, Rochat E, Martin E, Rochat S, Bula CJ. Instruments measuring spirituality in clinical research: a systematic review. *J Gen Intern Med*. 2011;26:1345–1357.

40. Draper P. An integrative review of spiritual assessment: implications for nursing management. *J Nurs Manag*. 2012;20:970–980.

41. Lunder U, Furlan M, Simonic A. Spiritual needs assessments and measurements. *Curr Opin Support Palliat Care*. 2011;5:273–278.

42. LeFavi RG, Wessels MH. Life review in pastoral care counseling: background and efficacy for the terminally Ill. *J Pastoral Care Council*. 2003;57:281–292.

43. Chochinov HM, Kristjanson LJ, Breitbart W, et al. Effect of dignity therapy on distress and end-of-life experience in terminally ill patients: a randomised controlled trial. *Lancet Oncol* 2011;12:753–762.

44. Taylor EJ. *What Do I Say? Talking With Patients About Spirituality*. Philadelphia, PA: Templeton Press; 2007.

45. Taylor, EJ, Mamier I. Spiritual care nursing: What cancer patients and family caregivers want. *J Adv Nurs* 2005;49(3):260–267.

46. Kvale K. Do cancer patients always want to talk about difficult emotions? A qualitative study of cancer inpatients communication needs. *Eur J Oncol Nurs*. 2007;11(4):320–327.

47. Taylor EJ. Client perspectives about nurse requisites for spiritual caregiving. *App Nurs Res*. 2007;20(1):44–46.

48. Ellis MR, Campbell JD. Patients' views about discussing spiritual issues with primary care physicians. *South Med J*. 2004;97:1158–1164.

49. Maugens TA. The SPIRITual history. *Arch Fam Med*. 1996;5:11–16.

50. Skalla KA, McCoy JP. Spiritual assessment of patients with cancer: the moral authority, vocational, aesthetic, social, and transcendent model. *Oncol Nurs Forum*. 2006;33:745–751.

51. Power J. Spiritual assessment: developing an assessment tool. *Nurs Older People.* 2006;18(2):16–18.

52. Pronk K. Role of the doctor in relieving spiritual distress at the end of life. *Am J Hospice Palliat Med.* 2005;22:419–425.

53. Byrne M. Spirituality in palliative care: what language do we need? Learning from pastoral care. *Int J Palliat Nurs.* 2007;13(3):118–121.

54. Rumbold BD. A review of spiritual assessment in health care practice. *Med J Austr.* 2007;186(10):S60–S62.

55. Timmins F, Kelly J. Spiritual assessment in intensive and cardiac care nursing. *Nurs Crit Care.* 2008;13(3):124–131.

56. Telos N. Proactive: spiritual care for terminal restlessness. *Palliat Support Care.* 2005;3:245–246.

57. Sexson SB. Religious and spiritual assessment of the child and adolescent. *Child Adolesc Psychiatr Clin N Am.* 2004;13:35–47.

58. Mueller CR. Spirituality in children: understanding and developing interventions. *Pediatr Nurs.* 2010;36:197–203, 208.

59. Heilferty CM. Spiritual development and the dying child: the pediatric nurse practitioner's role. *J Pediatr Health Care.* 2004;18:271–275.

60. Buck HG, McMillan SC. A psychometric analysis of the Spiritual Needs Inventory in informal caregivers of patients with cancer in hospice home care. *Oncol Nurs Forum.* 2012;39(4):E332–E339.

61. Delgado Guay MO, Parsons HA, Hui D, De la Cruz MG, Thorney S, Bruera E. Spirituality, religiosity, and spiritual pain among caregivers of patients with advanced cancer. *Am J Hosp Palliat Care.* 2012;30(5):455–461.

62. Barnes LP, Plotnikoff GA, Fox K, Pendleton S. Spirituality, religion, and pediatrics: intersecting worlds of healing. *Pediatrics.* 2000;104:899–908.

63. Ferrell B, Baird P. Deriving meaning and faith in caregiving. *Sem Oncol Nurs.* 2012;28:256–261.

64. Otis-Green S, Ferrell B, Borneman T, Puchalski C, Uman G, Garcia A. Integrating spiritual care within palliative care: an overview of nine demonstration projects. *J Palliat Med.* 2012;15:154–162.

65. Improving the quality of spiritual care as a dimension of palliative care. [Conference proceedings.] March 6–7, 2013; Los Angeles, CA.

66. Anandarajah G, Hight E. Spirituality and medical practice: using the HOPE questions as a practical tool for spiritual assessment. *Am Fam Physician.* 2001;63:81–89.

67. LaRocca-Pitts M. A spiritual history tool: FACT. Available at http://www.professionalchaplains.org/files/resources/reading_room/spiritual_history_tool_fact_larocca_pitts.pdf. Accessed March 31, 2015.

68. McEvoy M. An added dimension to the pediatric health maintenance visit: the spiritual history. *J Ped Health Care.* 2000;14:216–220.

Chapter 2

Spiritual Care Intervention

Rev. Pamela Baird

Spiritual care is, perhaps, the most mysterious and most often misunderstood part of palliative care. There is much discussion about what constitutes good spiritual care, and to date there is no agreed-upon definition. The misunderstanding is caused in part by this lack of agreement. To demystify spiritual care, it is important to establish clear definitions. For the purposes of this chapter, the terms are defined as follows:

- *Spirituality:* "Spirituality is the aspect of humanity that refers to the way individuals seek and express meaning."[1]

  "An organization that has a set of rites, rules, practices, values, and beliefs that prescribe how individuals should live their lives and "includes a relationship with a divine being."[2]

- *Spiritual Care:* Allowing our humanity to touch another's by providing presence, deep listening, empathy, and compassion.[3]

- *Compassion:* The ability to be empathetically present to another while he or she is suffering and trying to find meaning.[4,5]

- *Existential:* Relating to human existence and experience.[6]

Although the literature is trending toward defining the terms *spiritual* and *religious* differently, some authors use them interchangeably, implying they are the same. It is sometimes assumed that spiritual care is only about a person's religious traditions and beliefs. Using the definitions above, not everyone would describe himself or herself as religious, but everyone is spiritual.[1] In fact, these definitions can determine the care given to patients. If a person does not identify as religious and the spiritual care offered is only about religious issues, then the person has been denied care that could, in fact, provide compassion, peace, and comfort in the midst of the fear, pain, and chaos of illness. Much spiritual care can be given to support a person's relationship with himself or herself, others, nature, and the transcendent, even when religion is not a factor.

Spiritual Care Needs of Caregivers

A 65-year-old woman, dying of breast cancer, was being cared for by her husband and the hospice team. The couple had been married for 43 years, had no children, and at present had very few family members or friends to support them in her dying. The woman was attended by hospice for a couple of months before she died. She was lethargic, bed-bound, and slept many hours of the day. She said she didn't want or need to see a chaplain, but her husband did. The chaplain met the woman once very briefly to introduce herself, but after that, all visits concentrated on providing spiritual care to the husband, who despite his best efforts, was being overcome by anticipatory grief.

The husband was a retired navy cook. He was high energy, engaging, talkative, and very guarded when it came to feelings and emotions. He was eager for the chaplain's visits. He was of Italian heritage, raised in the Catholic Church, but was not a particularly religious person. Spiritual care for this man consisted of listening to his stories about cooking for the troops on a ship, stories about his life in the navy and with his wife, and feeding the chaplain. The first few visits, the chaplain tried diligently to avoid eating, not wanting to inconvenience the husband or cause him undue concern by thinking he had to feed her. But after a couple of visits where he insisted she sit down and eat, she realized that cooking for and feeding someone was just what he needed. His wife was no longer interested in food and certainly couldn't hold a conversation for very long. What he *knew* was cooking and feeding people, and now that his life was unraveling, he needed to engage in something pleasant and familiar that would help him cope with the grief he was trying so hard to ignore.

It was over the bowls of homemade soup that this husband, at times, felt safe enough to engage in some bits of conversation about his grief, his feelings, and his dying wife.

What Is Spiritual Care?

Spiritual care is simply meeting the other person human to human, providing compassionate presence, and being available for whatever comes up. In the case study in the previous section, not only was it unnecessary to talk about God, or anything religious, but it would have been inappropriate and perhaps off-putting. The spiritual interchange took place just by being with the person, understanding where he was—emotionally and spiritually—and taking care of what was important to him.[4]

At other times, with other people, spiritual care might include saying prayers, reading from holy texts, or talking about God and the mysteries of the universe. It is not for us to decide what the spiritual care looks like. On some level, what we do to provide spiritual care is less important than *who* we bring into the room. Good spiritual care requires that the person who walks into the room put aside his or her own expectations and agenda and, instead, focus on the patient—doing whatever is needed, at the time, for the person receiving the care.

At its core, spiritual care is about being honest, being authentically human, and allowing our own humanity to touch the humanity of another[7] (Box 2.1). In the course of offering spiritual care, God, religious beliefs, and ideas may emerge, but they do not have to. Religion is one way, one very important and significant way, that we express our spirituality. But religion is not a

Box 2.1 The Essential Elements of Spiritual Care

Spiritual care encompasses:

- Authenticity
- Kindness
- Compassion
- Respect
- Dignity
- Humanity
- Vulnerability
- Service
- Honesty
- Empathy

prerequisite. Spirituality can be expressed in a million ways: sitting quietly by the side of the road, taking food to a friend, watching a toddler learn to walk, working in the garden, praying, or crying with a man whose wife just died.

Rachel Naomi Remen speaks to the essence of spiritual care when she writes about the difference between "helping" and "serving." When we "help" someone, we assume they are broken and need fixing—they are weak, we are stronger, and we have the answers. But when we go to the bedside not to help or fix, but to serve, we allow our humanness, our wholeness, our brokenness, our compassion, and our vulnerability to be present and forefront. When we "help" or "fix" patients, they are in our debt. Service requires no payment. Service is mutually beneficial. When we serve, we create a space where healing can occur, both for the served and the server.[7]

"I'm Only the Nurse. What Do I Know About Providing Spiritual Care?"

Spiritual care is in the purview of everyone: the medical staff, the palliative care team, and the patient's family and friends.[1] Given the mystery and misunderstanding surrounding spiritual care, it is understandable that many people feel unqualified and uncomfortable providing spiritual interventions. Many feel

Box 2.2 Questions Requiring Chaplain Referral

- What have I done to deserve this?
- I pray, but I'm still sick.
- I used to believe in God, but now I'm not so sure.
- How will my family get along without me?
- What did my life mean?
- I'm scared.

> ### Box 2.3 Spiritual Interventions
>
> - Compassionate presence
> - Listening deeply
> - Bearing witness
> - Compassion at work

that because they, themselves, are not religious, they could not possibly be of spiritual support to anyone. Others, although defining themselves as religious, do not feel comfortable praying out loud or with someone else, or they think they do not know the Bible or the Quran, or any of the other holy books, well enough. Here again, the religious interventions are only a part of spiritual care, and they are often best handled by the chaplain or professional spiritual caregiver. If patients are asking questions about God, expressing concerns, or ruminating over existential issues, then an appropriate intervention would be to make a referral to the chaplain (Box 2.2).[1] Chaplains are trained to address spiritual and existential concerns, both religious and nonreligious. However, a chaplain referral is not the only spiritual intervention that can, or should, be made.

Because nurses are at the bedside 24/7 and, generally, are the medical professionals who spend the most time with patients and their families, it is important for them to know how to provide spiritual care and to do it well. It does not require a special degree, but it does take awareness of oneself, and the other, and it takes effort and a strong commitment. As stated earlier, at its core spiritual care is about being human and allowing our humanity to touch the humanity of another. Our humanity is expressed, in part, by providing presence, listening deeply, bearing witness, and putting our compassion into action.[8] This is the foundation of spiritual care (Box 2.3).[8]

Compassionate Presence and Deep Listening

It is not possible for the medical community to promise that a patient will never experience pain or suffering or to guarantee a calm and peaceful death. But it is possible to promise to accompany the patient on the journey. This does not mean that an individual nurse should promise to be at the patient's side always, but it does mean the medical team can assure the patient it will do everything possible to alleviate pain and suffering and that the patient and family will not be abandoned.[9]

Being present is much more than just being in the room. In the words of John H. Kearsley, "it is insufficient merely to be physically present. I have had to realize that to make my presence count . . . I need to be *really* present, psychologically and emotionally."[10] Psychological presence entails work and effort on the part of the caregiver. Kindness, deep listening, and empathy are required for psychological or compassionate presence.[11]

Providing compassionate presence is more than just showing up or walking into a room. There is a quality to the presence that gives the message, "There is nowhere else I would rather be at this moment than here with you." It is not just about being physically in the room with another, but being present in that room—body, mind, and spirit. It is about "exhibiting empathy and focused attention."[12,13] Presence does not take any more time than just showing up, but it does take a lot more effort, energy, and intention, and it makes an enormous difference to the recipient. A nurse can go into a patient's room, walk directly to the IV pole, hang the medication, turn, and walk out. Or, that same nurse can go into the patient's room, walk over to the patient, make eye contact, smile, gently touch the patient's hand, walk to the IV pole, hang the medication, look directly into the patient's eyes once again, smile, turn, and walk out the door.

Human beings have a need to be seen and heard. "When dying patients are seen, and know that they are seen, as being worthy of honor and esteem by those who care for them, dignity is more likely to be maintained."[14] Spiritual care is about preserving dignity and truly seeing the other person. It is also about hearing the spirit of the message. It is not enough just to see the body or to hear the words. Spiritual care is about connecting to the heart, mind, and soul because that connection says, "I see you. I hear your concerns. You matter. You are important. You are not alone. I care."

A woman and her family were going through hard times. There were children to feed, a mortgage, and all the usual expenses that go along with supporting a family of six. The woman and her husband owned a business that had been floundering for four years, and they were close to losing everything. They had $2.48 in the bank, creditors calling, and no guarantee of when more money would arrive. The woman was in her minister's office, embarrassed, telling her story, crying, and feeling terrified by life. As she was pouring her heart out, someone walked by the minister's door and caught the minister's attention. The minister immediately stood up and waved, said, "Oh, hello!" and began talking to the passerby. The parishioner never again shared anything of importance or consequence with her minister.

To listen deeply means hearing what is being said and what is not being said and trying to understand the emotions and feelings behind the words. It means to "tune in" to another person, so that we understand who that person really is on a deep, authentic level.[15] Listening deeply requires the ability to hold the pain and suffering of another. When someone trusts us enough to be vulnerable in our presence and then goes even further, explaining the circumstances of the pain and suffering, he or she has offered us a gift. It is our responsibility to embrace and protect that gift and treat it with the utmost respect, care, and deference.

The minister dismissed the woman's pain and trivialized her suffering by allowing herself to be distracted when being present was so crucial. It could have been a time of healing. Although the minister could not change the woman's circumstances, she had the opportunity to be truly present, thereby offering a human connection to the woman who was in such despair. The minister missed the moment and ensured that she would never again be given the chance to connect with her parishioner in such an intimate way.

Talking, listening, and telling our stories are all part of the human experience. In a study conducted by Mako, Galek, and Poppito to investigate spiritual pain, they found that patients were more likely to request that someone sit and talk and be with them than they were to ask for religious interventions. "Patients asked that the chaplain 'Stay with me as long as possible,' and 'Stop by every now and then and talk to me.'"[25] Listening deeply and being "psychologically" or compassionately present are spiritual interventions that anyone can learn. But it takes time, practice, effort, willingness, and intention to be truly available to another human being. Many patients receiving palliative care have been told that there is no cure for them. A cure may not be possible, but the opportunity for healing is. Healthcare professionals can be the conduit to healing simply by being present and listening deeply.

Bearing Witness

The term *bearing witness* may seem a foreign concept to some, but it is integral to spiritual care and a part of our experience as human beings. A friend is diagnosed with cancer, a coworker dies, an airplane crashes. These sad, life-changing events, and those that are happy and joyous as well, generally stimulate a response. That response is to tell the story of what happened. We feel the need to share our experiences, and we feel compelled to hear other people's stories. To bear witness is to be present to the events and the emotions of another's life and experience. We find strength and comfort in knowing that other human beings bear witness to the significant events of our lives—the good and the bad.

It may seem that bearing witness is a passive event, such as just watching and observing. But indeed, beneficially bearing witness takes focus and intention just as compassionate presence and deep listening do. Bearing witness is not "fixing," "helping," or imparting answers or platitudes. Platitudes are seldom healing and "answers" can function to alienate the one we seek to serve. People seek medical attention looking for answers. There are some things in medicine that have definitive answers and some that do not. In the spiritual/existential realm, there are very few, if any, absolutes. Two people asking the question, "Why did I get sick?" will most likely get two different answers, if they can find answers at all. Our spiritual/existential answers are our own, revealed to us through years of living life through our own lens and experience. Nurses and healthcare providers might find it a relief to know that they do not have to have the answers to patients' spiritual questions. Furthermore, offering an answer to another's spiritual questions, or providing meaning, is not in the purview of healthcare professionals and generally is not helpful or beneficial.[13] We cannot know the answers to others' questions, so to assume we do and to assert those "answers" might be harmful to the patient or, at the very least, impede their own process of finding meaning.

So what does it really mean to bear witness? Bearing witness means compassionate presence, deep listening, watching, observing—being with. "Your job is to offer not only compassion but also to accompany as best as you can those dying on their journey."[17] Bearing witness means to compassionately accompany another.

Like presence and listening, bearing witness does not mean taking away the person's pain or suffering. Bearing witness means being present to the pain and suffering. In fact, if our primary goal is to take away the suffering, then that itself can interfere with our ability to be present in the moment.[18] Bearing witness is the ability to sit in the midst of whatever is happening. We often betray our own discomfort while listening to the stories of patients' suffering, when we jump up to get a tissue for their tears. We tell ourselves that the tissue is for the one who is crying, to make him/her more comfortable, when in fact it may say more about our own desire to step back and move away from the pain. The message we risk sending is, "Stop crying. I don't want to hear any more. I need you to stop crying now."

When someone is sharing an intense story, if we are truly present in the moment, then we can find ourselves almost not breathing while we listen to or attend to the other. When we move, we break the moment, and it can stop the process, the story, and the tears. Something as simple as reaching over and touching a person, while he or she is telling the emotion-filled story, can stop the flow and interrupt the process. When these interruptions occur, there is a good chance that the story, which was so important to tell, might never again find the opportunity to be told. It takes time, experience, and thoughtful awareness to learn when to speak, or move, or get tissues.

Bearing witness means being comfortable enough in our own pain and suffering, that we can just sit quietly, be with another human being who is suffering, and not run. It also means being aware of our own grief, and being in touch with that grief, so that it does not spill over and leak out onto the patients and families we serve.

Managing Patient and Caregiver Grief

Mrs. S, a 42-year-old female patient with advanced ovarian cancer, was readmitted to the hospital experiencing severe nausea, vomiting, pain, and weight loss caused by a blockage in her intestines. She was weak, frightened, and very anxious. She was married with two children, whose ages were five and seven. This was the first time the medical staff who had been caring for her for the past five years could remember this patient exhibiting behavior of fear or anxiety. Her physician had the reputation of being uncomfortable with the "human" side of cancer. She would not address questions about a patient's mortality or inquiry of, "What will happen if the chemo doesn't work and the cancer keeps growing?" This oncologist would either ignore the question and move on to something else or would minimize her patient's concern with, "Now let's not worry about that. You just keep strong and keep doing what we tell you to do and you'll be fine."

Mrs. S, who had always acquiesced to her physician's will, was now unwilling to be dismissed, as her fear and anxiety escalated. The doctor was described as "cold," and some said "rude," when attempting to allay her patient's anxiety and agitation upon admission. The doctor, appearing upset and frustrated, gave an order for medication to sedate Mrs. S. The sedation was given for the next two days with the patient's agitation and anxiety returning each time the medication wore off.

The social worker and chaplain, who knew this woman well, discussed with each other the high likelihood that the reason for the anxiety was Mrs. S's desire to know what was really happening in her body, so she could plan for her family's future. Her husband and children were of paramount importance to her, and Mrs. S had discussed with the chaplain and the social worker, on more than one occasion, her desire to know what was likely to happen, so she could prepare her family. If she was going to die from this disease, she did not want it to be a surprise to everyone, especially her husband and children.

The social worker and chaplain each met with Mrs. S to assess her psychosocial and spiritual needs and concerns. They concurred that their primary intervention would be to ask Mrs. S what she thought was causing her anxiety and to carefully listen to what she had to say. She reported to both of them that she felt like she was going to die, and she just needed the doctor to tell her the truth. Both social worker and chaplain strongly encouraged the patient to tell her doctor that she wanted, and *needed*, to know what might happen to her.

The social worker and chaplain together spoke with the physician. They explained to the doctor that the patient's anxiety might be significantly decreased if she would sit and speak with Mrs. S and give her an honest prognosis. The doctor listened and somewhat reluctantly agreed, before saying how hard it is for her to lose a patient. She did not like the "dying part" of being a doctor.

After the physician and Mrs. S had a conversation about the patient's poor prognosis, the anxiety dramatically decreased, eliminating the need for sedation.

It is not easy for caregivers to manage both their own grief and the grief of their patients. But to ensure that professional caregivers are providing the best care for their patients and are caring for themselves as well, it is incumbent upon them to be aware of, work with, and reconcile their own grief.[19] This will be addressed more fully later in the chapter.

Compassion at Work

Being present, listening deeply, and bearing witness require a commitment from the one who serves. After these interventions, the next step in providing good spiritual care is action based on compassion. Is there anything missing? Is there something more to be done? Deep listening can reveal a patient's hopes, desires, and longing. Sometimes what is needed is very simple, but it can make a huge difference in the quality of the patient's life.

For many, healthcare professionals and laypersons alike, being unsure of what to say can cause discomfort at the thought of spending any quality time with one who is dying. Empathy is vital to spiritual care. The capacity to put ourselves in the place of another is paramount. We can never know what another person is really feeling, but we can, in our own mind, imagine what it might be like for us to be in the patient's situation: "How would I feel if I was the one who was dying?" "What would I want?" "What would I want someone to say . . . or not say?" "What would feel supportive?"

To ask ourselves these kinds of questions is the first step in being attuned to the other person's suffering and pain. Although we can only guess what a patient might or might not want to talk about, we can ask some open-ended, leading questions that will give the patient the opportunity to express his or her feelings, if he or she chooses. If we ask a question or two and the patient seems reticent or reluctant to talk, then we can assume that either this is not a good time, or it is not something he or she wants to talk about with us. It does not mean we never ask another question, but that we take our cues from the patient, listening carefully for a time when he or she might be open and willing to talk.

We often hear, for instance, "Mrs. White just does not want to talk about it." This may or may not be true. When we are experiencing pain and suffering, it is not uncommon for us to be very particular with whom we share our feelings and innermost thoughts. We want to make sure that the person we tell will have some understanding of what we are going through and will respect our feelings and care for them. So, although Mrs. White "does not want to talk about it" with just anyone, she might be willing, even eager, to talk if the right person walked into her room—a person who would listen deeply, be present, and bear witness to her deepest fears and concerns. This would likely be a person who would know when to honor the silence and say nothing and then would know what to say at the appropriate time.

How do we know what to say? This is something we can learn with time and experience. It is vital to be observant when we are with other people, listening to what they say, when they say it, and how the message is delivered. Watching to see what "works" and what "does not" can be a wonderful way for us to learn how to listen and communicate effectively, especially in sensitive circumstances. To learn this skill requires that we be acutely aware—aware of our own responses and the responses, verbal and nonverbal, of those people we are observing.

It is almost always appropriate to ask a person to tell us more about the story. "How did you feel when that happened?" "What happened next?" "Tell me more about that." There are times when we are so touched or overwhelmed by a story that we honestly do not know what to say. It is an authentic response and it is not inappropriate to say, "I have no idea what to say at this moment." Because it is genuine and honest, people usually respond well to a statement that bears such candor. It is certainly preferable to making a casual remark that runs the risk of trivializing the person's feelings or the situation.

Even when a person is open and wants to talk about his or her experience and feelings, it can be difficult to know just how far to take the conversation. What questions are appropriate to ask? Questions that inquire about a person's feelings or experience are generally welcomed (Box 2.4). If a question is asked that a patient does not want to answer, he or she usually will find a way to "talk around" the question without actually giving an answer. Listening carefully to what is "not" said is crucial. It can tell us that the patient, at this moment, does not want to go there.

Box 2.4 Spiritual Care Questions

Are you scared?

What makes life worth living?

Is there anything you haven't done that you need to do?

What do you hope for?

What are you most afraid of?

Is there anything worse than death?

What are you most proud of in your life?

Do you have regrets?

Sometimes talking and listening are not enough. What a patient has to say may reveal that he or she needs more: a chaplain referral, a phone call to a family member, prayer, a walk in the garden, or that he or she has a feeling of urgency to leave the hospital and go home. Just as advocating for patients is a standard component of nursing care, it is also a vital element of spiritual care and is a spiritual care intervention.

How Listening to Stories Provides Clues to Spiritual Needs

A 58-year-old single woman, with no children or close family members, was admitted to the hospital to receive a bone marrow transplant for the treatment of leukemia. The woman was fairly isolated, having only two or three friends who might visit during her hospital stay, which could last anywhere from weeks to months. When the chaplain went in to meet with the patient the first day, the woman did not identify herself as "religious" but did remark that being out in nature gave her a sense of connection to the universe, calmed her, and helped her to feel at ease. She spent most of her days outside in her garden and felt better there than anywhere else. She was wondering how she was going to survive being inside for the next few weeks. She told the chaplain she was feeling scared about the transplant and depressed at the thought of being cooped up inside unable to see her garden.

After hearing just how important nature was to her spiritual well-being, the chaplain noticed the room the woman had been given had a very large window, but it overlooked a freeway with nothing in view but thousands of cars and high-tension wires . . . no trees or flowers or anything that could be even loosely referred to as nature. The chaplain was very aware that the transplant unit was full; however, this was a real potential for spiritual distress and might easily be averted with a simple remedy. The opposite side of the unit also had large windows . . . that overlooked a beautiful mountain range with green trees and flowers and plants—nature at its finest! That afternoon, the chaplain met with the people who could make the room transfer possible. It was not easy convincing those who assigned the rooms that this change was not just, "Oh, I think it would be nice if she could have a pretty view while she's here," but rather a necessary spiritual intervention that could impact the patient's ability to cope and heal from the transplant. It took 3 days, but the change was made, and the woman was delighted that she could commune with nature during her transplant, in the comfort of her hospital bed.

Presence, deep listening, and bearing witness were important and vital, but in this case, more was needed. Sometimes just engaging in life review—telling the story of one's life—is what brings a sense of peace, and there is nothing more to be done. In other cases, it is not enough just to be with, be present, and listen. Sometimes, as with this patient, the situation calls for action, for doing something more.

Patients often give us specific information when we engage them in conversation, but it is not the only way we discover who patients are and what is important to them. Sometimes the clues are more subtle. They can be as simple as noticing a rosary on the bed or pictures of grandchildren on the wall. Sometimes just being aware of who visits the patient can provide insight about his or her spirituality. Noticing that a rabbi visited the patient can be a perfect entrée to asking about a person's spiritual or religious beliefs: "I noticed a rabbi came to see you this morning. It made me wonder if you're Jewish, and if you are, if there is anything we can do here in the hospital to support you in your faith?" It is important to ask and not just assume that because a rabbi was in the room that the person is Jewish. But it does give the healthcare provider a place to start, in an effort to determine what kind of spiritual care, if any, the person may want or need.

Below are some examples of discovering a patient's wants or needs:

- One man had been hospitalized for the better part of a year, and it had been extremely difficult for him and his family. He was a bone marrow transplant patient, which meant he could not have plants or flowers in his room and could not go outside for much of that year he was in the hospital. Only after the "spiritual intervention" from his daughter did the staff discover that he was quite a gifted rose gardener. It was somewhat ironic, because the hospital was known for its huge rose gardens. Unfortunately, not being allowed outside meant this patient was not able to enjoy them. However, his daughter had the idea of photographing the roses in his yard as well as some on the hospital grounds. She took beautiful, close-up pictures of individual roses in all stages of unfolding, had the prints enlarged, cut around each one of them, and taped those hundreds of roses all over the walls of his room. It was beautiful! It gave enjoyment to not only the patient and his family but to the medical staff, as well. Moreover, it revealed something significant about the man and generated conversation with him, as a person, apart from his identity as a patient. It made him more than just another body in a bed, with no particular identity other than his diagnosis. He was the one in the hospital who loved to be outside and knew how to grow beautiful roses. It gave the staff another way to connect with him, besides just his illness.

- A week before Christmas, the chaplain was paged back to the hospital shortly after leaving for the night. A 35-year-old patient was about a week away from dying and her mother and father, who were at her bedside, requested the chaplain come pray with them. The patient, who for medical reasons could no longer speak, was not particularly interested in a prayer, but she did want to sing Christmas carols. She couldn't make a sound to talk but was able to make a little noise when she tried to sing. The words were completely unintelligible, but some of the tune made itself known. The patient, her mother, and the chaplain sang for the better part of the evening, one carol after another, frequently joined by a nurse, phlebotomist, or other healthcare professional as they entered the room to give care. Before leaving for the night, the chaplain rushed out to buy Christmas CDs, which the family played all night, according to the parents' report the next day.

- An elderly woman, dying at home with hospice care, told the team that years before, she and her husband had raised English Setters. She spoke longingly about that time in their lives. The chaplain had a friend who had an English Setter. He and his dog, Sarah, were a part of the local hospital's pet team. Sarah was very comfortable being with people who were sick in bed. With the patient's and her husband's consent, the chaplain made arrangements for Sarah to visit and lie beside the woman in her last days. The pleasure and the memories were apparent on the patient's face as she hugged and petted Sarah.

Some patients clearly verbalize what they need physically, mentally, emotionally, and spiritually and are eager to talk and share their feelings. Yet others just do not express who they are, and what they need, quite so obviously, try as we might to help them. But when we do discover something that will provide comfort, or a way for a person to more fully express his or her spirituality, it is important to do whatever we can to make it available. The clues, and the outcomes, do not have to be dramatic. One patient told everyone who would listen about her favorite nurse. The reason the nurse was so special? Whenever she went into the room to provide care, she sang the patient a song. These signs are merely ways to start a conversation about what is meaningful in a person's life.

The nurse does not have to be the only one to provide spiritual interventions. He or she may be the one to learn what is needed, but sometimes another member of the healthcare team might be better suited to make it happen. If a patient wants someone to come and pray, perhaps the chaplain would be the best person to provide the intervention. If the patient's goal is to complete a will or advance directive, then maybe the social worker would be best to call. Sometimes it takes more than one person to help the patient achieve his or her goal. For example, a nurse discovers that the patient does not want further medical treatment and really just wants to go home to die. The nurse offers spiritual intervention when she advocates for the patient by informing the physician and the medical team, who make it possible for the patient to leave the hospital.

Spiritual care means finding a way to make a connection, discovering any needs or desires that might improve quality of life, and then advocating and making arrangements for the fulfillment of those needs and desires. The job of a spiritual caregiver is always to be open (absent an agenda), listen, observe, and, when in doubt, ask questions. Assuming anything without asking leaves open the possibility that we will get it wrong. We never can be certain what is inside someone else's mind and heart. To ask is always best.[20]

The Use of Rituals in Spiritual Care

Often, when we think of rituals, we speak of religious traditions that have been practiced and passed down for hundreds or thousands of years. Some of the most obvious rituals are Holy Communion; Anointing of the Sick; prayer; Scripture reading, chanting, and singing; or saying the rosary.

But rituals do not have to be religious in nature. They can be created spontaneously, in the moment, to meaningfully acknowledge a person, event, or circumstance in our lives. Angeles Arrien stated, "Ritual is recognizing a life change, and doing something to honor and support the change."[21] We engage in nonreligious, yet spiritual, rituals everyday: when we bake a birthday cake for a friend and sing "Happy Birthday," read a bedtime story to our children each night, or even read the newspaper over a cup of coffee in the morning.

When patients are receiving palliative care, they have often been sick for a long time and sometimes forget who they were before the illness began. Many times, the disease becomes the descriptor by which they identify themselves. For patients to avoid losing their identity to the disease, it can be especially helpful to maintain as much normalcy as possible, particularly when they have been confined to the hospital for long periods of time. Birthday cakes, bedtime stories, and reading the morning paper with a cup of coffee are simple rituals that can remind them of what they held dear, before the onset of the disease.

In a cancer hospital where bone marrow transplants require patients to be hospitalized for weeks—even months—at a time, a group of patients created a ritual that served them well. Every evening after dinner, they met in a lounge area and played cards. This ritual was the highlight of their hospital stay. They looked forward to an activity that, under normal circumstances, might seem ordinary and routine. But here this ritual afforded them the opportunity to not only get out of their rooms, but also to be with other people (who also had a good understanding of what they were going through), to forget they had cancer for awhile, to participate in an activity that felt normal again, to socially engage with other people ... and the list goes on. The nursing staff was incredibly supportive, adjusting the schedules of what needed to be done, so that these patients could be free in the evenings to participate in their nightly ritual.

Nurses can be invaluable in suggesting and supporting such rituals for patients. When professional caregivers are aware of their patients as unique individuals with distinct wants, needs, and desires, they can offer meaningful suggestions for rituals that might support the patient's life and experience. Listening to music during unpleasant treatments might be soothing to a musician or a teenager who loves music. Getting a patient dressed early each morning, before breakfast, might help that person feel more able to take on the day. Sitting at the bedside to hear a patient's stories could be important to a young mother who wants to talk about the time she spent with her children who visited earlier in the day. The list of rituals is endless.

Although religious rituals are fewer in number, they can be equally important and beneficial. Caregivers cannot be expected to know all the religious rituals people practice, so it can be beneficial for the nurse, and others, to ask patients about any traditions or rituals that may be meaningful or important to them. Although the healthcare professional may not be involved with the rituals themselves, they can play a vital role in making sure the patient has some time alone, uninterrupted, so that the ritual will have the opportunity to be fully expressed and experienced.

Rituals are a part of each of our lives. By recognizing the importance of ritual and by facilitating their expression, nurses can be the conduit through which palliative care patients can find support and meaning.

Spiritual Care Near the Time of Death

As death draws near, it is even more important that professional caregivers attend to patients and their families with kindness, authenticity, and deep awareness. This awareness hears what is being said and not said, and sees the visual signs of want, need, desire, and distress. Even those families who cannot begin to entertain the possibility of death are aware, on some level, that life is changing. So it is a great kindness to be especially insightful and responsive to their wants, needs, desires, feelings, and fears. Patients may not be able or willing to ask for what they want, but if nurses and other healthcare professionals are attentive and perceptive, clues are frequently obvious and reveal what is needed. When providing spiritual care for those who are imminently dying, the three most important things to remember are: don't wait; intently watch and listen; and trust your instincts.

A grandmother, who was in relatively good health until three weeks prior, fell and broke a hip, was bedridden at home, on hospice, and declining rapidly. Some days she was alert and oriented; other days, she was wildly confused. This particular Friday morning began with her mind and memory cloudy. While sleeping, her breathing pattern changed and it caught the attention of her granddaughter. The elderly woman was being cared for around the clock by her three daughters and a granddaughter who also worked as a hospice chaplain. Becoming aware of the subtle changes, the granddaughter instinctively felt they should call the rest of the family to the bedside. They did just that, and within a couple of hours, there were dozens of grandchildren, great-grandchildren, family members, and friends assembled in the old woman's tiny house.

When the family began to arrive, the grandmother perked up and became much more alive and alert than she had been in weeks. This woman, who loved her family deeply but was never one to hug or kiss or show affection of any kind—and certainly had never been described as having a sense of humor—blossomed and came to life in front of her family. She was affectionate, chatty, warm, and funny, and her family saw a side of her no one there had ever witnessed in the grandmother's 90 years. The day was filled with stories and great humor. She lived another 10 days. They were quiet days, and she was withdrawn and frequently confused. Although the family never again experienced the joy, affection, and laughter of that Friday, family members continue to describe it as the best time they ever had with the grandmother, and they are exceedingly grateful for the gift. Had the granddaughter ignored the almost imperceptible signs of decline and neglected to call in the family, who knows if they ever would have had another opportunity to experience their loved one in such a significant way?

It is easy to doubt and question ourselves or dismiss signs and clues that are often barely visible and unclear. Good spiritual care, especially for the dying, requires caregivers to hone their skills in assessing these subtleties. Don't wait; intently watch and listen; and trust your instincts. To not do these things risks missing the moment and the opportunity that, literally, might never come again for the one who is dying.

Healthcare Professional Grief, and Well-Being

Every day, healthcare professionals deal with their patients' grief, but that does not make the caregivers immune to their own. The death of a loved one or friend is not the only kind of grief we experience. All people who are alive and aware experience grief, whether or not they have ever known someone who has died. When someone is disrespectful and rude to us, when we do not get the job we want, or when we are transferred to another part of the country, we experience grief. Grief can be the belief that we are not enough or that we failed, or the realization that life is changing, and our hopes and dreams will never be realized.[32] When a loved one dies or when we experience extreme disappointment and loss, the grief never completely goes away, but with time and effort, it is possible to come to terms with the loss, establish a new relationship with the deceased or the circumstance, and move on.[22]

Although time does have its own way of easing suffering, it is not the only thing required to heal our grief. Grief is not an event. Grief is not linear. It is a process and it takes not only time, but effort, energy, work, and intention. It is most often a sequence of "two steps forward, one step back." Individual grief therapy or grief support groups can be useful tools in teaching us how to deal with our grief.

It is also important for us to be patient and have mercy for ourselves[23] There is no set time frame for grief. It takes as long as it takes. One man whose wife died felt it took him about three years to reconcile the loss. Another husband felt like he hadn't moved forward at all, even five years after his wife died.

Many hospices, which have served to educate our society on the importance of the grief process, give their employees only three days' paid bereavement—and then only for very immediate family members. Very often the person has not been buried, or a service conducted, in those three days, and the shock of the death can delay active grieving for some time. Three days is not enough time to face the world after a painful loss and then be expected to act as though everything is just fine. Just being familiar with death and grief does not guarantee understanding, or ease, in dealing with the process. Healthcare professionals can have just as much difficulty as their patients—maybe more—given the frequency with which they come face to face with dying, death, and grief. It can be difficult to care for someone who is grieving, when the caregiver is in the midst of his/her own grief journey. A caregiver's grief can be triggered just by being in the presence of a patient who is also grieving. It is sometimes challenging for a busy caregiver to distinguish between the patient's grief and his or her own. For the well-being of all concerned, it is essential for healthcare professionals to be aware of and deal with their own grief and loss. Nurses and others are better able to serve when they have acknowledged their own pain and have made the effort to work through their own grief process.[24]

Conclusion: Nurses Providing Spiritual Care

Although deep listening, presence, bearing witness, and compassion are all simple ideas, these interventions are not easy. To provide them in a way that invites healing requires from the caregiver, a willingness to learn, the ability to be without agenda, and the commitment to be ever vigilant and self-introspective. Nurses, who are often called upon to provide these interventions, are at the forefront of patient care. They are asked every day to deal with the medical, emotional, social, and spiritual crises and burdens of others' lives. They are expected to ease suffering whenever and wherever possible. At best, nursing is difficult work. We seem to be asking almost superhuman acts from nurses, who deeply want to provide all that is asked of them. Fortunately, quality spiritual care does not require superhuman acts—just human kindness, compassion, and caring.

References

1. Puchalski C, Ferrell B, Virani R, et al. Improving the quality of spiritual care as a dimension of palliative care: the report of the consensus conference. *J Palliat Med.* 2009;12(10):885–904.

2. Puchalski C, Ferrell B. *Making Health Care Whole: Integrating Spirituality*. West Conshohocken, PA: Templeton Press; 2010.

3. McSherry W, Ross L. Nursing. In: Cobb M, Puchalski CM, Rumbold B, eds. *Oxford Textbook of Spirituality in Healthcare*. New York, NY: Oxford University Press; 2012:211–217.

4. Bryson KA. Spirituality, meaning, and transcendence. *J Palliat Support Care.* 2004;2:321–328.

5. Post SG. *Unlimited Love: Altruism, Compassion and Service*. Philadelphia, PA: Templeton Foundation Press; 2003.

6. Existential, definition and synonyms. Macmillian Dictionary Web site. www.macmillandictionary.com/dictionary/american/existential. Accessed June 20, 2013.

7. Remen RN. In the service of life. *Noetic Sci Rev.* 1996;37(Spring):24–25.

8. Halifax J. *Project on Being With Dying Training for Health Care Professionals*. Upaya Zen Center Web site. Santa Fe, NM: 2001. http://www.upaya.org/being-with-dying/articles-writings/. Accessed April 13, 2015.

9. Sulmasy DP. Ethical principles for spiritual care. In: Cobb M, Puchalski CM, Rumbold B., eds. *Oxford Textbook of Spirituality in Healthcare*. New York, NY: Oxford University Press; 2012:465–470.

10. Kearsley, JH. Wal's story: reflections on presence. *J Clin Oncol.* 2012;30(18):2283–2285.

11. Neff KD. Self-compassion: an alternative conceptualization of a healthy attitude toward oneself. *Self Identity.* 2003;2:85–102.

12. McDonough-Means S, Kreitzer MJ, Bell I. Fostering a healing presence and investigating its mediators. *J Altern Complement Med.* 2004;10(S1):S-25–S-41.

13. Guenther MB. Healing: the power of presence. A reflection. *J Pain Symptom Manage.* 2011;41(3):650–654.

14. Chochinov HM, Cann BJ. Interventions to enhance the spiritual aspects of dying. *J Palliat Med.* 2005;8(S-1):S-103–S-115.

15. Slater V. What does "spiritual care" now mean to palliative care? *Eur J Palliat Care.* 2007;14(1):32–34.

16. Mako C, Galek K, Poppito SR. Spiritual pain among patients with advanced cancer in palliative care. *J Palliat Med.* 2006;9(5):1106–1113.

17. Halifax J. Personal communication, December 12, 2008.

18. Millspaugh D. Assessment and response to spiritual pain: Part II. *J Palliat Med.* 2005;8(6):1110–1117.

19. Ferrell BR, Baird P. Deriving meaning and faith in caregiving. *Semin Oncol Nurs.* 2012;28(4):256–261.

20. Pronk K. Role of the doctor in relieving spiritual distress at the end of life. *Am J Hosp Palliat Med.* 2005;22(6):419–425.

21. Arrien A. *The Four-fold Way.* San Francisco, CA: Harper San Francisco; 1993.

22. Klaus D, Silverman PR, Nickman SL. *Continuing Bonds: New Understandings of Grief.* Philadelphia, PA: Taylor & Francis, 1996.

23. Levine S, Levine O. *The Grief Process.* Boulder, CO: Sounds True; 1999.

24. Feldstein CBD. Bridging with the sacred; reflection of an MD chaplain. *J Pain Symptom Manage.* 2011;42(1):155.

Chapter 3

Cultural Considerations in Palliative Care

Polly Mazanec and Joan T. Panke

This chapter defines culture and the complexity of its components as they relate to palliative care, emphasizing that one's own values, practices, and beliefs impact care. This is not intended to be a "cookbook" approach to describing behaviors and practices of different cultures as they relate to palliative care, but rather a guide to raising awareness of the significance of cultural considerations in palliative care.

Culture and Palliative Care Nursing

The essence of palliative nursing is to provide holistic supportive care for the patient and the family living with a serious or life-limiting illness. Palliative nursing strives to meet the physical, emotional, social, and spiritual needs of the patient and family across the disease trajectory.[1] To meet these needs, nurses must recognize the vital role that culture has on the experience of living and dying. The beliefs, norms, and practices of an individual's cultural heritage guide one's behavioral responses, decision-making, and actions.[2] Culture shapes how an individual makes meaning out of illness, suffering, and death.[2,3] Nurses, along with other members of the interdisciplinary team, partner with the patient and family to ensure that the patient's and family's values, beliefs, and practices guide the plan of care.[4]

The National Consensus Project for Quality Palliative Care's Clinical Practice Guidelines[4] define the core concepts and structures for quality palliative care delivery. Eight domains with corresponding criteria reflect the depth and breadth of the specialty. Cultural aspects of care are identified as one of the eight domains, emphasizing the central role that culture plays in providing strength and meaning for patients and families facing serious illness.[4] Within this domain, culture is defined and cultural competence for interdisciplinary team members is outlined in two overarching guidelines, as well as its clinical implications (see Box 3.1).

Culture is a source of resilience for patients and families and plays an important role in the provision of palliative care. It is the responsibility of all members of the palliative care program to strive for cultural and linguistic competence to ensure that appropriate and relevant services are provided to patients and families. The following case illustrates the distress experienced

Box 3.1 Clinical Practice Guidelines for Quality Palliative Care—Cultural Aspects of Care

Guideline 6.1: The palliative care program serves each patient, family, and community in a culturally and linguistically appropriate manner

Criteria:

- Definition of culture and cultural components
- Cultural identification of patient/family
- Assessment and documentation of cultural aspects of care
- The plan of care addresses the patient's and family's cultural concerns and needs
- Respect for the patient's/family's cultural perceptions, preferences, and practices
- Palliative care program staff communicates in a language and manner that the patient and family understand and takes into account:
  - Literacy;
  - Use of professional interpreter services and acceptable alternatives;
  - Written materials that facilitate patient/family understanding.
- Respects and accommodates dietary and ritual practices of patients/ families.
- Palliative care staff members identify and refer patients/families to community resources as appropriate.

Guideline 6.2: The palliative care program strives to enhance its cultural and linguistic competence

Criteria:

- Definition of cultural competence;
- Valuing diversity in the work environment. Hiring practices of the palliative care program reflect the cultural and linguistic diversity of the community it serves.
- Palliative care staff cultivate cultural self-awareness and recognize how their own cultural values, beliefs, biases, and practices inform their perceptions of patients, families, and colleagues.
- Provision of education to help staff members increase their cross-cultural knowledge and skills, and reduce health disparities;
- The palliative care program regularly evaluates and, if needed, modifies services, policies, and procedures to maximize its cultural and linguistic accessibility and responsiveness. Input from patients, families and community stakeholders is integrated into this process.

Adapted from National Consensus Project for Quality Palliative Care. Clinical Practice Guidelines for Quality Palliative Care. 3rd ed. Pittsburgh, PA: National Consensus Project for Quality Palliative Care; 2013. http://www.nationalconsensusproject.org/Guidelines_Download2.aspx.

by the patient, family, and healthcare team when cultural implications of care are not considered.

Case Study

Mrs. S is a 79-year-old female admitted to the hospital with decompensated congestive heart failure. She and her husband moved to the United States from China in the early 1970s and raised a daughter and son in the United States. Her 85-year-old husband is in good health. On morning rounds, the medical team spoke to the patient about her diagnosis, prognosis, likely disease course, and advance care planning concerns, without any other family present. The palliative care service was consulted in the afternoon to assist the primary team, after the nurse found Mrs. S's husband helping her dress and stating he was taking her to another hospital that would respect their ways.

Questions to Consider in This Case Are:

1. What cultural issues are likely the basis for the conflict between the husband and medical team?
2. What cultural, religious, and/or spiritual issues might impact decision-making?
3. Who might the palliative team involve to assist in ascertaining religious or cultural aspects of care?
4. What are some techniques that the nurse and other health providers might use to both respect the patient's right to be involved in his or her care and ascertain what she wants to know and who will make decisions for this patient?

Increasing Diversity in the US Population

As the United States becomes increasingly diverse, the range of treasured beliefs, shared teachings, norms, customs, and languages challenges nurses to understand and respond to a wide variety of perspectives. The total US population mid-2013 was estimated to be 313.9 million and is projected to cross the 400 million mark by 2051.[5] Population statistics from the US Census Bureau illustrate that cultural diversity is increasing among the most common racial groups, which are federally defined as American Indian/Alaskan Native, Asian/Pacific Islander, Black or African American, and White (Table 3.1).[6] The Hispanic population is categorized in the census statistics as an ethnic group, not a racial group.

In 2012, the fastest-growing racial group was Asians, with more than 60% of the growth stemming from international migration. By comparison, Hispanics represent the second fastest-growing and second largest population in the United States, behind non-Hispanic whites, with their population increase mostly related to birth rate. Rates of growth in 2012 for other groups include: Native Hawaiians and Other Pacific Islanders, increase of 2.2% to about 1.4 million; American Indians and Alaska Natives, a rise of 5% to a little over 6.3 million; and Blacks or African Americans, increasing 1.3% to 44.5 million.[7]

Table 3.1 Ethnic Groups, Census 2012	
White	197.7 million
Hispanic	53 million
Black or African American	44.5 million
Asian	18.9 million
American Indian/Alaskan Native	6.3 million
Hawaiian & Other Pacific Islanders	1.4 million

Data from Humes KR, Jones NA, Ramirez RR. Overview of race and Hispanic origin: 2010. 2010 Census briefs. Washington, DC: United States Census Bureau; March 2011. www.census.gov/prod/cen2010/briefs/c2010br-02.pdf. Accessed June 23, 2013.

Census projections in 2012 suggest that by 2060, the combined minority groups, which currently make up 37% of the US population, will become the majority (57%).[5] Diversity among age groups is also changing as the population ages. By 2060, citizens 65 years and older will more than double and the "oldest old," the 85-years-and-older age group, is expected to more than triple between 2012 and 2060.[5] It is quite probable that intergroup diversity will also increase, adding to the complexity of culturally competent care and the potential for cultural clashes.

With changes in cultural diversity in the US population comes increasing diversity in the nursing workforce. Nurses must be aware of how one's own cultural beliefs and norms shape professional practice and differ from the beliefs and norms of patients and families for whom they care.

Culture Defined

Culture is the "learned, shared and transmitted values, beliefs, norms and life ways of a particular group that guide their thinking, decision, actions in patterned ways—a patterned behavioral response."[8] Culture is shaped over time in a dynamic system in which beliefs, values, and lifestyle patterns pass from one generation to another.[3] This dynamic organizing system of life is adaptive, designed to ensure survival and well-being and to find a common purpose or meaning throughout life.[3]

Although culture is often mistakenly thought of as simply race and ethnicity, the definition of culture is multidimensional, encompassing such components as gender, age, differing abilities, sexual orientation and identity, religion, and socioeconomic factors (financial status, residency, employment, and educational level).[2] Each cultural component plays a role in shaping individual responses to life and, in particular, to serious illness and death.[2,3]

A broad definition of culture recognizes the various subcultures with which an individual may associate, that shape experiences and responses in any given situation. The nurse must be aware constantly that the culture of the healthcare system and nursing profession, as well as personal beliefs, shape how he or she responds in patients', families', and colleagues' interactions.

Components of Culture

Race

The commonly held misconception that *race* refers to biological and genetic differences and *ethnicity* refers to cultural variation is outmoded. Race exists not as a natural category, but as a social construct.[9] Any discussion of race must include the harsh reality of racism issues and disparities that have plagued society and continue to exist even today. Recent studies have demonstrated the discrimination against persons of certain races regarding healthcare practices, treatment options, and hospice utilization.[10–13] When viewed in relation to specific races, morbidity and mortality statistics point to serious gaps in access to quality care. Racial disparities are still evident, even after adjustments for socioeconomic status and other access-related factors are taken into account.[14]

One factor that may contribute to racial disparities in healthcare is the underlying mistrust of the healthcare system many individuals of certain racial backgrounds have, because of terrible injustices of the past. Memories of the Tuskegee syphilis study and segregated hospitals remain with older African Americans.[15] The combination of mistrust and numerous other complex variables influence palliative care issues, such as medical decision-making and advance care planning, which require a trusting relationship between patient and provider.[3,16] Compounding the situation is the fact that healthcare providers often do not recognize existing biases within systems or themselves.[14,17] These unknown biases may add to the perceived discrimination experienced.[14,17,18]

Ethnicity

Ethnicity refers to "a group of people that share a common and distinctive racial, national, religious, linguistic, or cultural heritage."[18] The values, practices, and beliefs that members of the same ethnic group share may influence behavior or response. Ethnicity has been identified as a significant predictor of end of life preferences, decision-making, and disparities in access to quality care.[19] Currently, there are more than 100 ethnic groups and more than 500 American Indian Nations in the United States.[18]

Ethnicity has been shown to influence utilization of hospice and palliative care services. Ethnic minority groups are less likely to use hospice services when compared to non-Hispanic whites. Furthermore, there has been little increase in hospice utilization in black, Hispanic, or Asian populations in recent years.[16,20] Researchers have demonstrated the existence of disparities in quality end of life care among certain ethnicities, but have not yet identified why this is happening.[12] Evans & Ume (2012) recommend using a conceptual framework such as that used in the *National Healthcare Disparities Report* to explore causal mechanisms beyond race and ethnicity, which include access to care, receipt of care, quality of care, and examination of barriers; usage and costs of care; and effectiveness, safety, timeliness, and patient centeredness. Further utilization studies are needed.[21]

It is important to note that although an individual may belong to a particular racial or ethnic group, he or she may not identify strongly with that group.[2,8]

Members of the same family from the same ethnic group may have very different ideas about what is acceptable practice concerning important palliative care concepts, such as communication with healthcare professionals, medical decision-making, and end of life rituals. In multigenerational families, some members may hold to traditional beliefs and practices of their ethnic community of origin. Other family members may have a bicultural orientation, moving between the family culture of origin to the host society, and others may have left their cultural roots and identify with the host society.[22] For example, in the United States, second and third generations of immigrant families may be more assimilated into Western culture than the first generation, which can lead to cultural conflicts around sensitive palliative care concepts.

The tendency to assume that an individual will respond in a certain way because he or she is a member of an ethnic group contributes to stereotyping and can lead to inappropriate interventions and unnecessary distress. The nurse should assess each individual's beliefs and practices, rather than assuming that he or she holds the beliefs of a particular group. Note that many studies have demonstrated that, regardless of race or ethnicity, all persons share common needs at the end of life: being comfortable, being cared for, having sustaining or healing relationships, having hope, and honoring spiritual beliefs.[22–25]

Gender

Cultural norms dictate specific roles for men and women. The significance of gender is evident in palliative care areas such as decision-making, caregiving, and pain and symptom management. It is important to be aware of family dominance patterns and determine which family member or members hold that dominant role. In some families, decision-making may be the responsibility of the male head of the family or eldest son; in others, it may be the eldest woman. For example, those of Asian ethnicity who follow strict Confucian teaching believe that men have absolute authority and are responsible for family decision-making.[26] Discussing prognosis and treatment with a female family member is likely to increase family burden and distress and may result in significant clashes with the healthcare team.[2]

In addition to decision-making, cultural expectations exist regarding caregiving responsibilities. For many families, women traditionally have been expected to take on the role of caregiver when a family member is facing serious illness. In addition to work and childcare responsibilities, this added responsibility has been overwhelming for many, affecting their physical and emotional well-being. Research has demonstrated that female caregivers tend to experience greater caregiver burden, anxiety, and depression than male caregivers.[27,28] Family support of caregivers is an essential component of palliative care.

Age

Age has its own identity and culture.[2] Age cohorts are characterized by consumer behaviors, leisure and religious activities, education, and labor force participation. Each group has its own beliefs, attitudes, and practices, influenced by their developmental stage and society in which they live.[2] The impact of a life-limiting illness on persons of differing age groups is often influenced by the loss of developmental tasks associated with that age group.[29] As the US population ages, the importance of addressing elders' unique needs becomes more evident. Consider also the cultural impact of this aging population on cumulative loss, caregiving issues, medical decision-making, healthcare resources, and end of life choices.

Myths about the impact of age on pain management continue to exist, with some professionals believing that children and older adults do not perceive pain as strongly as other age groups. These beliefs result in pain undertreatment and unnecessary patient suffering in these vulnerable age groups.[30,31]

Differing Abilities

Individuals with physical disabilities or mental illness are at risk of receiving poorer quality healthcare. Those with differing abilities constitute a cultural group in themselves and often feel stigmatized. This discrimination is evident in cultures where the healthy are more valued than the physically, emotionally, or intellectually challenged.[2] If patients are unable to communicate their needs, then pain and symptom management and end of life wishes are not likely to be addressed. Additionally, this vulnerable population's losses may not be recognized or acknowledged, putting individuals at risk for complicated grief. Challenges to providing palliative care and hospice services to those with intellectual disabilities include the fact that residential facility providers have limited palliative care knowledge and may need to increase their knowledge about caring for patients with intellectual disabilities.[32] Taking time to determine an individual's goals of care—regardless of differing abilities—and identifying resources and support to improve quality of life is essential.

Sexual Orientation and Identity

Sexual orientation may carry a stigma when the patient is gay, lesbian, bisexual, or transgender. In palliative care, these patients have unique needs, because of the legal and ethical issues of domestic partnerships, multiple losses that may have been experienced as a result of one's sexual orientation, and unresolved family issues. Domestic partnerships, which are sanctioned by many cities and states in the United States, grant some of the rights of traditional married couples to unmarried homosexual couples who share the traditional family bond.[2] However, other cities and states do not legally recognize this relationship. A durable power of attorney for healthcare must be completed. Without such documentation, decision-making follows state guidelines. If legal documents have not been drafted prior to a partner's death, then survivorship issues, financial concerns, and lack of acknowledgment of bereavement needs may cause additional distress and complicate grief.[33,34]

Unresolved family issues can complicate advanced illness stages and the dying process. The patient who is gay, lesbian, bisexual, or transgender may have been estranged from his/her family of origin. As the patient prepares for the end of life, reconciliation with family, old friends, or children may be desired; it may be challenging and distressing when family dynamics prohibit this healing opportunity.[32]

Religion and Spirituality

Religion is the belief and practice of a faith tradition, a means of expressing spirituality. Spirituality, a much broader concept, is the life force that transcends our physical being and gives meaning and purpose.[29] Although religion and spirituality are complementary concepts, these terms should not be used interchangeably. Note that an individual may be very spiritual but not practice a formal religion. In addition, those who identify themselves as belonging to a religion may not necessarily adhere to all the religion's practices. As with ethnicity, it is important to determine how strongly the individual aligns with his or her identified faith and its practice rituals.

Religious beliefs can significantly influence a person's decisions regarding treatment and care. These beliefs can be at the cornerstone of decisions regarding continuation or discontinuation of life-prolonging therapies for some people.[10] Additionally, religious beliefs can strongly influence how patients and families understand illness and suffering.[3,10]

Chaplains—clergy from a patient's or family member's religious group, ideally their own community clergy—are key members of the interdisciplinary palliative care team. Those who turn to their faith-based communities may find the emotional, spiritual, and other tangible support they need when dealing with a serious or life-limiting illness.[12,19,24] Keep in mind, however, that some individuals who are struggling with misconceptions of their own faith's tenets may experience spiritual distress and need spiritual intervention from caring chaplains or spiritual care counselors. Also be aware that community clergy may not have specific end of life care training, and may need assistance from the palliative care team to support the patient's spiritual journey.

Spirituality is in the essence of every human being. It is what gives each person a sense of being, meaning, purpose, and direction.[35,36] It transcends the self to connect with others and with a higher power, independent of organized religion.[12,29,35] One's sense of spirituality is often the force that helps transcend loss and suffering.[24,25,29] Spiritual distress can cause pain and suffering, if not identified and addressed. Assessing spiritual well-being and attending to spiritual needs, which may be very diverse, is essential to quality of life for patients and families confronting end of life.

Socioeconomic Status

One's socioeconomic status, place of residence, workplace, and level of education are important components of one's cultural identity and play a role in palliative care. For example, those who are socioeconomically disadvantaged face unique challenges when seeking healthcare and receiving treatment. Expenses—including pain medications, medical tests, treatments, and drugs not covered by limited insurance plans; transportation; and childcare—add additional burdens. It is important to note, however, that regardless of financial status, an estimated 25% of families are financially devastated by a serious terminal illness.[2] Patients experiencing disease progression, or in whom treatment side effects preclude the ability to work, are forced to confront profound losses: of work and income, of identity, and of a colleague network.

Those who are educationally disadvantaged struggle to navigate the healthcare system and to find information and support—especially needed when dealing with a serious illness. The educationally disadvantaged may lack knowledge about resources, such as palliative care services, and may not have the skills or access to the global Internet and social networking.

Access to services is challenging for some depending on their geographic location. For those living in rural areas, access to palliative care services is inadequate when compared to those in urban areas.[37] Only 57% of public hospitals, which serve those without health insurance or those in rural areas, provide palliative care services.[38] Hospice services are also lacking, with 62% to 92% of rural counties in selected states reporting no access to community-based hospice services.[39] Patients and families in a supportive community have increased access to resources at end of life compared to other, more vulnerable populations.[2]

A very vulnerable population with limited community resources is that of unauthorized immigrants. It is estimated that there are about 11.5 million unauthorized immigrants in the United States,[40] most of whom are educationally and socioeconomically disadvantaged and living without healthcare. Most unauthorized immigrant care is emergent only; little is known about access to palliative and hospice care in this population.

Conducting a Cultural Assessment

Many tools are available to help with cultural assessment. Posing questions and obtaining answers in a cultural assessment requires development of the patient's/family's trust. When meeting the patient and family early in the disease trajectory, the palliative care nurse often has the advantage of time to establish such a relationship—but not always. Using the skills of presence and active listening is often more beneficial than using a standardized tool. Checklists do not necessarily build trust and can be burdensome. Simple inquiries into patient and family practices and beliefs can assist the nurse in understanding needs and goals. Asking the patient and/or the family member to talk about themselves or the family and then listening to those narratives is powerful. The patient and family often give clues that trigger important questions that can clarify their needs and goals. Box 3.2 provides examples of trigger questions.

Box 3.2 Key Cultural Assessment Questions

Formal cultural assessments are available for the nurse to use. Remember that a checklist does not always instill trust. Below are some suggestions for ascertaining key cultural preferences from both patients and family caregivers.

- Tell me a little bit about yourself (e.g., your family, your mother, father, siblings, etc.).
- Where were you born and raised? (If an immigrant, "How long have you lived in this country?")
- What language would you prefer to speak?
- Is it easier to write things down, or do you have difficulty with reading and writing?

(continued)

Box 3.2 (Continued)

- To whom do you go for support (family friends, community, or religious or community leaders)?
- Is there anyone we should contact to come to be with you?
- I want to be sure I'm giving you all the information you need. What do you want to know about your condition? To whom should I speak about your care?
- Who do you want to know about your condition?
- How are decisions about healthcare made in your family? Should I speak directly with you, or is there someone else with whom I should be discussing decisions?
- (*Address to patient or designated decision-maker*) Tell me about your understanding of what has been happening up to this point? What does the illness mean to you?
- We want to work with you to be sure you are getting the best care possible and that we are meeting all your needs. Is there anything we should know about any customs or practices that are important to include in your care?
- Many people have shared that it is very important to include spirituality or religion in their care. Is this something that is important for you? Our chaplain can help contact anyone that you would like to be involved with your care.
- We want to make sure we respect how you prefer to be addressed, including how we should act. Is there anything we should avoid? Is it appropriate for you to have male and female caregivers?
- Are there any foods you would like or that you should avoid?
- Do you have any concerns about how to pay for care, medications, or other services?

Death Rituals and Practices

- Is there anything we should know about care of the body, about rituals, practices, or ceremonies that should be performed?
- What is your belief about what happens after death?
- Is there a way for us to plan for anything you might need both at the time of death and afterward?
- Is there anything we should know about whether a man or a woman should be caring for the body after death?
- Should the family be involved in the care of the body?

Selected Palliative Care Issues Influenced by Culture

Communication

Communication is the foundation for all encounters between healthcare providers, patients, and family members.[41] When the providers and the patient–family unit are from different ethnic or cultural backgrounds, relating news regarding serious illness or a poor prognosis can be challenging. Communication disparities may lead to poorer outcomes and reduced patient and family satisfaction.[3,42] Increasing diversity in the US population challenges clinicians to gain competency in cultural aspects of communication. Each individual brings his or her own cultural experiences, and assumptions about the world, health, and illness, to each new encounter, and it is important to assess and respect differing viewpoints.[9,23] The establishment of a relationship with the clinician, where he or she seeks to understand the patient's and family's individual concerns, provides a foundation for all future communication and decision-making.[22,45]

Communication is an interactive, multidimensional process, often dictated by cultural norms; it provides the mechanism for human interaction and connection. Given the complexities of communicating diagnosis, prognosis, and progression of a life-limiting disease, there is no "one size fits all" approach.[43] Cultural assessments, including cultural norms related to communication, should occur early in the initial assessment; findings should be clearly documented and shared with all providers involved in the care of the patient and family.

General communication principles should be utilized at all times. These include (1) adequate preparation for communicating medical facts; (2) selecting a private setting, free from distractions; (3) using appropriate nonverbal communication styles, such as sitting down, maintaining eye contact, and conveying that the clinician is not rushed; and (4) expressing empathy and responding to patient and family emotional responses.[43]

One of the most important cultural communication assessments involves determining how information is shared within the family unit. Determine who the decision-maker is, whether it is the patient or a specific family member or members, and with whom information should be shared. For example, relating a diagnosis or poor prognosis to the patient may go against some cultural norms. Ideally, preferences for communication, including full disclosure of a terminal diagnosis and poor prognosis, are best discussed early in the clinician–patient relationship, when the patient is relatively healthy. When this is not possible, clinicians should take time to reflect on their own bias, listen to patient and family concerns, determine individual and group norms, and engage in an ongoing dialogue about such preferences. Such measures will strengthen the relationship and show respect for the unique ways in which a family group functions.[44,45]

Determine the dominant language and dialect spoken and the literacy level of both the patient and the family. If there is a language barrier, a professionally trained interpreter of the appropriate gender should be contacted. If such services are not available, healthcare providers, ideally trained in palliative care, may serve as interpreters. Family members should only act as interpreters in emergency situations, and only if they agree to do so, since family members placed in this role may feel uncomfortable should sensitive issues or questions arise.[4] Always determine what is culturally appropriate to disclose prior to discussion, regardless of who is involved in the communication of medical information.[3] When using an interpreter, direct all verbal communication to the patient or family rather than the interpreter. Ongoing clarification that information is understood is critical.

Active listening is one of the most important communication techniques for the palliative care nurse to master. Elicit patient and family concerns, customs, norms, beliefs, and values, and take time to reflect back what is heard. Encourage patients and families to also reflect back what they have heard. Listening to words alone is not enough. Pay attention to nonverbal cues (e.g., gestures, posture, use or avoidance of eye contact). Nonverbal communication will give valuable information and insight into the emotional impact of what is being said, and will help inform the clinician regarding how to behave as well. Additional communication skills are described in Box 3.3.

Medical Decision-Making

Over the past 45 years in the United States, ethical and legal considerations of decision-making have focused on patient autonomy.[10,19] This focus has replaced the more paternalistic approach of decision-making as solely the physician's responsibility with an approach that emphasizes a model of shared responsibility with the patient's active involvement.[16] The Patient Self-Determination Act of 1991 sought to clarify and protect an individual's healthcare preferences with advance directives.[46] The principle of respect for patient autonomy points to a patient's right to participate in decisions about the care he or she receives. Associated with this is the right to be informed of diagnosis, prognosis, and the risks and benefits of treatment to make informed decisions. Inherent in the patient autonomy movement is the underlying assumption that all patients want control over their healthcare decisions. Yet, in fact, for some individuals, patient autonomy may violate the very principles of dignity and integrity it proposes to uphold and may result in significant distress.[3,10]

This European American model of patient autonomy has its origin in the dominant culture, a predominantly white, middle-class perspective that does not consider diverse cultural perspectives.[3] In fact, in some cultures, patient autonomy may not be viewed as empowering, but rather as isolating and burdensome for patients who are too sick to make difficult decisions.[3,10]

Emphasis on autonomy as the guiding principle assumes that the individual, rather than the family or other social group, is the appropriate decision-maker.[43] However, in many non–European American cultures, the concept of interdependence among family and community members is valued more than individual autonomy.[3,10,19] Cultures that practice family-centered decision-making, such as the Korean American culture, may prefer that the family, or perhaps a particular family member, rather than the patient, receives and processes information.[10,12] For example, the traditional Chinese concept of "filial piety" requires that children, especially the eldest son, are obligated to respect, care for, and protect their parents.[47] Based on this culture's values and beliefs, the son is obligated to protect the parent from the worry of a terminal prognosis.

Although full disclosure may not be appropriate, it is never appropriate to lie to the patient. If the patient does not wish to receive information and/or giving it to the patient violates the patient's and family's cultural norms, the

Box 3.3 Culturally Competent Communication Skills and Best Practices for Palliative Care Clinicians

1. **Respect.** Baseline assessment and documentation should include primary language/dialect; determine need for professional interpreter services. Determine who is involved in giving/receiving information and decisions and how individuals prefer to be addressed.

2. **Person-centered interviews through active and reflective listening**. Hearing, understanding, retaining, analyzing, and evaluating information. Use information gleaned to guide future questions. Do not ask too many questions. Demonstrate active listening through an open body posture, eye contact (if culturally appropriate), and provide a private setting that is conducive to open communication. Reflect and restate essential content and determine other questions or concerns. Reaffirm intent to honor and respect individual/groups decisions and plans.

3. **Presence:** Know your own beliefs, values and your level of comfort in engaging in conversations regarding illness and distress. Assist individuals to meet realistic goals when facing a serious illness, challenging situation, and/or uncertain future. Listen to the stories, life goals, and values. Pay attention to interpretation time; for example, how long it takes to make decisions, time needed to complete individual goals, imminence of death. Show empathy and compassion; be quiet/reflective during times of silence.

4. **Clinical knowledge of disease trajectories.** Assess and address distressing symptoms, side effects of treatment, and likely disease progression. Reaffirm goals of care and attempt the relief of symptoms and other concerns. Incorporate preferred healing practices and traditions. Discuss early access to hospice care to support goals as disease progresses.

5. **Determine learning styles and provide education to patient and family.** Determine any deficits. Provide educational materials in preferred language and/or arrange for professional interpreter when providing education.

6. **Address nonverbal communication.**

7. **Assess the individual's interpretation of what is important in life, what gives life meaning for them.**

8. Spirituality

9. Privacy, boundaries, decision-making, loss, and grief

10. Anticipate times when communication will be difficult

Based on Long CO. Ten best practices to enhance culturally competent communication in palliative care. *Pediatr Hematol Oncol.* 2011;33(suppl 2):S136–S139.

healthcare provider who does so may not be respecting the patient's right to autonomously decide not to receive the information. Some cultures believe that telling the patient he or she has a terminal illness strips away any and all hope, causes needless suffering, and may indeed hasten death.[10,23] For example, imposing negative information, such as prognosis of a life-limiting illness, on the person who is ill is a dangerous violation of traditional Navajo values.[10]

The nurse must consider the harm that may occur when the healthcare system or providers violate cultural beliefs and practices. Assessing and clarifying the patient's and family's perspectives, values, and practices may prevent a cultural conflict.[2,45] The nurse is in a key position to advocate these critical patient and family issues. Box 3.2 provides examples of questions to ask during the assessment. By asking how decisions are made and whether the patient wishes to be told information or participate in the decision-making process, the healthcare team respects and honors patient autonomy, individual beliefs, and values.[45]

Discontinuation of Life-Prolonging Therapies

Another issue with the potential for cultural conflict surrounds decision-making on discontinuing or withholding life-sustaining treatments. Inherent in the decision is that the patient will most likely die. Attitude surveys evaluating initiating and terminating life-prolonging therapies have demonstrated several ethnic-group differences. Groups such as African Americans, Chinese Americans, Filipino Americans, Korean Americans, and Mexican Americans were more likely to start and continue such therapies than were European Americans, when the healthcare team felt such measures to be futile.[10,19,47,48]

Family members often feel that by agreeing to withdraw life-prolonging therapies, they are, in fact, responsible for the death of their loved one. For families who believe that it is the duty of children to honor, respect, and care for their elders, they may feel obligated to continue futile life-sustaining interventions. Allowing a parent to die may violate the principles of filial piety and bring shame and disgrace on the family.[47]

Religious beliefs may also play a role in the complexity of withholding or withdrawing medical interventions. For example, in the Christian Philippines, removing the ventilator is synonymous with euthanasia.[19] In Orthodox Judaism, where all life is valued as precious, only God can decide the time to die, and family members who agree to withdraw life-prolonging therapies may violate the patient's beliefs.[49] In both examples, involving a priest or rabbi may help the family and the healthcare team integrate religious tenets into the culturally appropriate plan of care.

A shared decision-making conversation emphasizing goals of care, rather than "medical futility," may help the family struggling with discontinuing life-prolonging therapies.[19,41] Recognize also that the words the healthcare team uses in presenting these decisions, including "do not resuscitate" and "withdrawal of life support," all have negative connotations and involve the removing of something or the withholding of a particular intervention. Words and phrases that may seem clear to the healthcare professional often get literally lost in translation, regardless of whether the parties speak the same language. "Withdrawal of life support" may be easily confused with stopping all care, which is not the intention. Feelings of abandoning or "giving up on the patient" can result from misinterpretation, creating family suffering, isolation, and distress.[23] The nurse is encouraged to be acutely aware of how information and/or questions are phrased. A suggestion is to use words that convey benefit versus burden of all therapies. Always begin the conversation with what the team will do to care for the patient, rather than what burdensome interventions should be stopped. Because many ethical conflicts arise from differences in patients', families', and providers' values, beliefs, and practices, it is critical that individual members of the healthcare team be aware of their own cultural beliefs, understand their own reactions to the issue, and be knowledgeable about the patients' and families' beliefs to address the conflict.[2]

Meaning of Food and Nutrition

Across cultures, there is agreement that food is essential for life to maintain body function and to produce energy. Food serves another purpose in the building and maintaining of human relationships. It is used in rituals, celebrations, and rites of passage to establish and maintain social and cultural relationships with families, friends, and others. Culturally appropriate foods may be used to improve health by groups who have strong beliefs about particular foods and their relationship to health.[26] Because of food's importance for life and life events, a loss of desire for food and subsequent weight loss and wasting can cause suffering for both the patient and family.

Families often need clear guidance and explanations for when a patient is no longer able to enjoy favorite foods or family mealtime rituals because of declining physical ability. Families often struggle when the patient ceases to consume nourishment or fluids, fearing that the patient will "starve to death" or suffer from dehydration. It is imperative that the healthcare team understand the meaning attached to food and nutrition, when decisions regarding the potential burden of providing artificial nutrition and hydration for an imminently dying patient are discussed. Exploring alternative ways in which the family can care for the patient through physical, spiritual, or emotional support will allow families to interact with the patient in ways that are meaningful to them and reflect individual beliefs, values, and preferences. The Hospice and Palliative Nurses Association Position Statement on Artificial Nutrition and Hydration in Advanced Illness can assist the nurse in understanding the benefits and burdens associated with this medical intervention.[50]

Pain and Symptom Management

Pain is a highly personal and subjective experience. Pain is whatever the person says it is and exists whenever the person says it does.[51] Culture plays a role in both the experience and meaning of pain and responses to it. The biopsychosocial model suggests that pain perception and response is influenced by biological, psychological, social, and cultural factors.[17] The meaning of pain varies among cultural groups. For some, pain is a positive response that demonstrates the body's ability to fight against disease or the dying process. For others, pain signifies punishment, and its value lies in the patient's ability to withstand the suffering and work toward resolution and peace.[17]

Strong beliefs about expressing pain and expected pain behaviors exist in every culture.[48] Pain tolerance varies from person to person and is influenced by factors such as past experiences with pain, coping skills, motivation to endure pain, and energy level. Western society appears to value individuals who exhibit a high pain threshold. As a result, those with a lower threshold, who report pain often, may be labeled as "difficult patients."

Pain assessment should be culturally appropriate, using terms that describe pain intensity across most cultural groups. *Pain, hurt,* and *ache* are words commonly used across cultures. These words may reflect the severity of the pain, with *pain* being the most severe, *hurt* being moderate pain, and *ache* being the least severe.[2] The healthcare team should focus on the words the patient uses to describe pain. To understand the severity of the pain of someone who does not speak English, the providers should use pain-rating scales that have been translated into numerous languages.[51] Although it is important to base the assessment on the patient's self-report of pain intensity, it may be necessary to rely on nonverbal pain indicators, such as facial expression, body movement, and vocalization, to assess pain in the nonspeaking cognitively impaired patient, the older adult, or the infant, who are all at risk for inaccurate assessment and undertreatment of pain.[2,51]

Racial, ethnic, age, and gender biases in pain management have been identified and documented. Studies of gender variations in pain response have identified differences in sensitivity and tolerance to pain, as well as the willingness to report pain.[30,52] Compared with men, women are more likely to report pain than men and have a lower pain threshold and tolerance in experimental settings.[52] Underidentification and undertreatment of pain is a well-recognized phenomenon in elder care.[53] Studies reveal that Hispanics, African Americans, and female patients are less likely to be prescribed opioids for pain or may be more unable to fill opioid prescriptions, depending on community access to pharmacies.[17]

Like pain, symptoms that patients receiving palliative care describe may have meanings associated with them that reflect cultural values, beliefs, and practices. Assessment and management of symptoms such as fatigue, dyspnea, depression, nausea and vomiting, and anorexia/cachexia should be addressed within a cultural framework. For example, some cultural groups may be hesitant to disclose depression, because it is considered a sign of weakness; instead, it may be referred to as a "tired state." Using culturally appropriate language, the nurse will need to evaluate whether the symptom experienced is fatigue or depression.

Incorporating culturally appropriate nondrug therapies may improve the ability to alleviate pain and symptoms. Herbal remedies, acupuncture, and folk medicines should be incorporated into the plan of care, if desired and safe. Keep in mind that certain nondrug approaches, such as hypnosis and massage, may be inappropriate in some cultures.

Death Rituals and Mourning Practices

Across all cultures, the loss of a loved one brings sadness and upheaval in the family structure.[48] Every culture responds to these losses through specific rituals that assist the dying and the bereaved through the final transition from life. It is important to note that rituals may begin before death and last for months or even years after death. Respecting these rituals and customs will have tremendous impact on the family members' healing process following the death and leave a positive lasting memory of the loved one's end of life experience. The nurse should make sure that any required spiritual, religious, or cultural practices are known, so that there is appropriate care of the body after death.

For example, dying at home is especially important for Hmong American elders who follow traditional beliefs.[54] The nurse in an acute care setting can be the advocate to ensure this tradition is honored. The family may consult a shaman to perform a ceremony to negotiate with the "God of the sky" to extend life. Additional ceremonies follow. Request for an autopsy or organ donation at the time of death is inappropriate because of the belief that altering the body will delay reincarnation. After the death, there is often much wailing and caressing of the body. The family prepares for an elaborate funeral with rituals to ensure that the loved one will "cross over" and continues with ceremonies for days following the funeral to make sure the soul joins its ancestors.[54]

The tasks of grieving are universal: to accept the reality of the loss, to experience pain of grief, to begin the adjustment to new social and family roles, and to withdraw emotional energy from the dead individual and turn it over to those who are alive.[55] The expressions of grief, however, may vary significantly among cultures. What is acceptable in one culture may seem unacceptable, or even maladaptive, in another. Recognizing normal grief behavior (vs. complicated grief) within a cultural context therefore demands knowledge about culturally acceptable expressions of grief.[2,55]

Case Study

Mr. M is a 62-year-old Vietnam War veteran who came to the Veterans Administration medical center for evaluation of cough, fatigue, weight loss, and pain in his right hip. He had not sought medical care for these symptoms, which had been going on for over three months. The outpatient oncology team was consulted for a new diagnosis of stage IV non–small-cell lung cancer, at the same time the palliative care service was called to assist with his care. Despite increasing pain in his hip and later, in his chest wall, he refused any pain medication other than ibuprofen. He repeatedly stated, "I am a tough Marine, I can take it, this is nothing compared to what some of my buddies went through in Nam." He confided in the chaplain that, "I deserve this, after all the people I hurt and killed in the war—this is payback." His anxiety and depressive symptoms worsened as the disease progressed. His wife and adult daughters were extremely distressed witnessing his suffering.

Questions to Consider in This Case Are:

1. What cultural issues may be contributing to the challenges of pain and symptom management for Mr. M?

2. What spiritual issues need to be addressed for a peaceful death?

3. What are some techniques that the nurse and other healthcare providers might use to help the family, as well as the staff, with moral distress surrounding poor pain management?

As you consider these questions, keep in mind the complex and often previously unresolved issues that surface for some of our veterans, when they are confronted with a serious, life-threatening illness. Veterans have their own unique culture, which is often specific to their branch of service and where they served. Understanding their military history and service experiences are an important part of a complete cultural assessment.[57,58]

Striving for Cultural Competence

Palliative care nurses value the importance of being culturally sensitive and striving for cultural competence. This sensitivity and competence is critical, when working with patients with a life-limiting illness and their families.

Cultural competence refers to a dynamic, fluid, continuous process of awareness, knowledge, skill, interaction, and sensitivity.[56] The term remains controversial, as some question whether one can ever become culturally competent.[3] However, cultural competence is an ongoing process, not an endpoint or something to be mastered.[22] It is more comprehensive than cultural sensitivity, implying not only the ability to recognize and respect cultural differences, but also to intervene appropriately and effectively. According to Campinha-Bacote's model for enhancing cultural competence, there are five components essential in pursuing cultural competence: cultural awareness, cultural knowledge, cultural skill, cultural encounter, and cultural desire.[56]

Integrating cultural considerations into palliative care requires, first and foremost, that the nurse become aware of how one's own values, practices, and beliefs influence care. Cultural awareness begins with an examination of one's own heritage, family practices, experiences, and religious or spiritual beliefs.[56] Because culture is a dynamic concept, it is important to reassess one's own beliefs on a regular basis, reflecting on beliefs that may have changed with increasing knowledge and cultural encounters.

Each nurse brings his or her own cultural and philosophical views, education, religion, spirituality, and life experiences to the care of the patient and family. The first component, cultural awareness, challenges the nurse to look beyond his or her ethnocentric view of the world, asking the question, "How are my values, beliefs, and practices different from the patient's and family's?" rather than, "How is this patient and family different from me?" Exploring one's own beliefs will raise an awareness of differences that have the potential to foster prejudice and discrimination and limit the effectiveness of care.[2,45] Exploring answers to the same cultural assessment questions used for patients and families increases self-awareness (Box 3.2). Often, this exploration identifies more similarities than differences. The universal aspects of life, family, trust, love, hope, understanding, and caring unite us all.

Acquiring knowledge about different cultural groups is the second component to striving for cultural competence, but knowledge alone is insufficient to provide culturally appropriate care.[56] No one can expect to have in-depth knowledge of all cultural variations of health and illness beliefs, values, and norms. A suggested strategy is to identify the most common ethnic groups and cultures living in the nurse's community and to integrate a basic understanding of norms and practices impacting issues likely to arise in palliative and end of life situations. To strengthen knowledge, one should seek out community members, organizations, faith communities, and leaders in a shared understanding of needs and concerns.

It is important to be aware that knowledge of a particular group should serve only as a guide to understanding the unique cultural needs of the patient and family, which comes through individualized assessments. Other resources, such as cultural guides, literature, and web-based resources, are available to assist the nurse in acquiring knowledge about specific groups. Box 3.4 lists several useful Web-based resources. It is important to remember that relying on culturally specific knowledge to guide practice, rather than individual assessment, is incongruent with culturally competent care.

Box 3.4 Web Resources for Acquiring Knowledge About Cultural Issues Affecting Healthcare

Cross Cultural Health Care Program (CCHCP): www.xculture.org
CCHCP addresses broad cultural issues that impact the health of individuals and families in ethnic minority communities. Its mission is to serve as a bridge between communities and healthcare institutions.

Diversity Rx: http://www.diversityrx.org
This is a great networking website that models and practices policy, legal issues, and links to other resources.

EthnoMed: http://ethnomed.org/
The EthnoMed site contains information about cultural beliefs, medical issues, and other related issues pertinent to the healthcare of recent immigrants to the United States.

Fast Fact & Concept #78: Cultural Aspects of Pain Management: https://www.capc.org/fast-facts/216-asking-about-cultural-beliefs-palliative-care/
This website contains many "fast facts" regarding palliative care. Number 78 addresses important cultural considerations and provides assessment questions when working with patients in pain.

Fast Fact & Concept # 216: Asking about Cultural Beliefs in Palliative Care: https://www.capc.org/fast-facts/216-asking-about-cultural-beliefs-palliative-care/
This resource offers a framework for assessing patient and family cultural needs by taking a "cultural history."

Office of Minority Health: https://minorityhealth.hhs.gov
This website has training tools for developing cultural competency.

Transcultural Nursing Society: http://www.tcns.org
The society (founded in 1974) serves as a forum to promote, advance, and disseminate transcultural nursing knowledge worldwide.

Cultural skill is the third component of cultural competency.[56] Cultural assessment, cross-cultural communication, cultural interpretation, and appropriate intervention skills can be learned. Multiple tools are available to assess cultural behavior and beliefs. For the new nurse, key assessment questions, applicable in the palliative care setting, may be helpful in guiding the assessment (Box 3.2). However, nothing can replace sitting with the patient and family and asking them to share their heritage/family history and cherished practices and beliefs.

The fourth component encompasses the concept of cultural encounters. Individuals with different ways of relating often misunderstand each other's cues. The more opportunities we have to engage with persons of different values, practices, and beliefs, the more we learn about others and ourselves, and the less likely we are to draw erroneous conclusions about each other. Active engagement with community leaders and use of learning tools such as case studies and role plays help expose nurses to varied cultural experiences.[56] Increasing exposure to cultural encounters may also improve confidence in one's ability to meet the needs of diverse populations.[56]

The fifth and final component of Camphina-Bacote's model for cultural competence is cultural desire. This is the interest and openness with which the nurse strives to understand patients and families and the communities from which they come. Cultural desire is the motivation to "want to" engage in the process of cultural competence, as opposed to being "forced to" participate in the process. The desire is genuine and authentic and encourages the nurse to take advantage of cultural encounters and explore worlds beyond his or her own ethnocentric perspective. Such experiences present opportunities for the nurse to grow both personally and professionally.[56]

Some researchers propose that the term *cultural humility* is more acceptable than cultural sensitivity or cultural competence when trying to provide culturally appropriate care.[59] Research suggests that multiple generations of blended families and intercultural marriages have made it nearly impossible to know all about healthcare practices of particular communities. These social scientists and writers recommend that nurses strive mindfully to respect each patient and family member as a unique individual rather than the components of culture (ethnicity, religion/spirituality, place of residence, etc.) that might label them.[22] We believe that integrating into clinical practice the proposed cultural competence model with cultural humility will strengthen nurses' ability to respect and support patient and family wishes in palliative care settings.

Summary

Given the changing population of the United States, we, as nurses, must advocate for the integration of cultural considerations in providing comprehensive palliative care. It is imperative that each of us move beyond our own ethnocentric views of the world to appreciate and respect one another's similarities and differences. We are challenged to embrace a better understanding of various perspectives. Striving for cultural competence first requires an awareness of how one's own cultural background impacts care. In addition, acquiring knowledge about cultures and developing skill in cultural assessment and communication are essential to improving palliative care for patients with life-limiting illnesses and their families. Most importantly, maintaining a sense of cultural humility, caring for each patient and family member as a unique human being with unique needs, and attending to their needs with dignity and respectfulness, is the essence of providing culturally sensitive care.

This chapter encourages nurses to integrate cultural assessment and culturally appropriate interventions into palliative care. It is the authors' hope that readers will enrich their practice by seeking knowledge about different cultures and, above all, by respectfully interacting with the most valuable resources on cultural considerations we have—our patients and their families.

References

1. Coyle N. Introduction to palliative nursing care. In: Ferrell BR, Coyle N, eds. *Oxford Textbook of Palliative Nursing*. 3rd ed. New York, NY: Oxford University Press; 2010:3–12.

2. American Association of Colleges of Nursing. End-of-Life Nursing Education Consortium (ELNEC) Web site. http://www.aacn.nche.edu/elnec/. Accessed June 23, 2013.

3. Kagawa-Singer M. Impact of culture on health outcomes. *Pediatr Hematol Oncol*. 2011;33(suppl 2):S90–S95.

4. National Consensus Project for Quality Palliative Care. *Clinical Practice Guidelines for Quality Palliative Care*. 3rd ed. Pittsburgh, PA: National Consensus Project for Quality Palliative Care; 2013.

5. Census Bureau projects U.S. Population of 315.1 million on New Year's Day [news release]. Washington, DC: United States Census Bureau; Dec. 27, 2012. https://www.census.gov/newsroom/releases/archives/population/cb12-255.html. Accessed June 27, 2013.

6. U.S. Census Bureau Projections show a slower growing, older, more diverse nation a half century from now [news release]. Washington, DC: United States Census Bureau; December 12, 2010. https://www.census.gov/newsroom/releases/archives/population/cb12-243.html. Accessed June 27, 2013.

7. Asians fastest-growing race or ethnic group in 2012, Census Bureau reports [news release]. Washington, DC: United States Census Bureau; June 13, 2013. http://www.census.gov/newsroom/releases/archives/population/cb13-112.html. Accessed June 27, 2013.

8. Leininger M. Quality of life from a transcultural nursing perspective. *Nurs Sci Quart*. 1994;7:22–28.

9. Koffman J, Crawley L. Ethnic and cultural aspects of palliative care. In: Hanks G, Cherney NI, Christakis NA, Fallon M, Kaasa S, Portenoy RK, eds. *Oxford Textbook of Palliative Medicine*, 4th ed. New York, NY: Oxford University Press; 2011:141–150.

10. Johnstone MJ, Kanitsaki O. Ethics and advance care planning in a culturally diverse society. *J Transcult Nurs*. 2009;20:405–416. doi:10.1177/1043659609340803.

11. Cohen LL. Racial/ethnic disparities in hospice care: A systematic review. *J Palliat Med*. 2008;5:763–767.

12. Evans BC, Ebere U. Psychosocial, cultural, and spiritual health disparities in end-of-life and palliative care: where we are and where we need to go. *Nursing Outlook* 2012;60:370–375.

13. Hulme PA. Cultural considerations in evidence-based practice. *J Transcult Nurs.* 2010;21:271–280. doi:10.1177/1043659609358782.

14. Smedley B, Stith A, Nelson A. *Unequal Treatment: Confronting Racial and Ethnic Disparities in Health Care (Report of the Institute of Medicine).* Washington, DC: National Academy Press; 2003.

15. Brandon DT, Isaac LA, LaVeist TA. The legacy of Tuskegee and trust in medical care: is Tuskegee responsible for race differences in mistrust of medical care? *J Natl Med Assoc.* 2005;97:951–956.

16. Bullock K. The influence of culture on end-of-life decision making. *J Soc Work End-of-Life Palliat Care.* 2011;7:83–98.

17. Anderson KC, Green CR, Payne R. Racial and ethnic disparities in pain: causes and consequences of unequal care. *J Pain* 2009;10:1187–1204.

18. The Office of Minority Health. National Center on Minority Health and Health Disparities Web site. http://www.ncmhd.nih.gov. Accessed June 29, 2013.

19. Manalo, MF. End-of-life decisions about withholding or withdrawing therapy: medical, ethical, and religio-cultural considerations. *Palliat Care: Res Treatment.* 2013;7:1–5. doi:10.4137/PCRT.S10796.

20. Mazanec PM, Daly BJ, Townsend A. Hospice utilization and end-of-life decision making of African Americans. *Am J Hospice Palliat Med.* 2010;27(8):560.

21. National Institute of Nursing Research. *The Science of Compassion: Future Directions in End-of-Life and Palliative Care* (Executive Summary). Bethesda, MD: National Institute of Nursing Research; 2011. https://www.ninr.nih.gov/sites/www.ninr.nih.gov/files/science-of-compassion-executive-summary.pdf. Accessed June 28, 2012.

22. Wittenberg-Lyles E, Goldsmith J, Ferrell BR, Ragan SL. *Communication in Palliative Nursing.* New York, NY: Oxford University Press; 2012;59–92.

23. Long CO. Ten best practices to enhance culturally competent communication in palliative care. *Pediatr Hematol Oncol.* 2011;33(suppl 2):S136–S139.

24. Prince-Paul MJ. Relationships among communicative acts, social well-being, and spiritual well-being on the quality of life at the end of life in patients with cancer enrolled in hospice. *J Palliat Med.* 2008;11:20–25.

25. Ferrell B, Coyle N. *The Nature of Suffering and the Goals of Nursing.* New York, NY: Oxford University Press; 2008.

26. Spector R. *Cultural Care: Guides to Heritage Assessment and Health Traditions.* 7th ed. Upper Saddle River, NJ: Pearson Education; 2009.

27. Northouse L, Williams A, Given B, McCorkle R. Psychosocial care for the caregivers of patients with cancer. *J Clin Onc.* 2012;30(11):1227–1234.

28. Otis-Green S, Juarez G. Enhancing the social well-being of family caregivers. *Sem Onc Nurs.* 2012;28(4):246–255.

29. Sherman DW. Culture and spiritual domains of quality palliative care. In: Matzo M, Sherman DW, eds. *Palliative Care Nursing: Quality Care to the End of Life.* 3rd ed. New York, NY: Springer; 2010:3–38.

30. Krok JL, Baker TA, McMillan SC. Age differences in the presence of pain and psychological distress in younger and older cancer patients. *J Hospice Palliat Nurs.* 2013;15:107–113. doi:10.1097/NJH.0b013e31826bfb63.

31. Soltow D, Given BA, Given CW. Relationship between age and symptoms of pain and fatigue in adults undergoing treatment for cancer. *Cancer Nurs.* 2010;33(4):296–303.

32. Stein, GL. Providing palliative care to people with intellectual disabilities: services, staff knowledge, and challenges. *J Palliat Med.* 2008;11:1241–1249. doi:10.1089/jpm.2008.0130.

33. Rawlings D. End-of-life care considerations for gay, lesbian, bisexual, and transgender individuals. *Int J Palliat Nurs.* 2012;18:29–34.

34. Higgins A, Glacken M. Sculpting the distress: easing or exacerbating the grief experience of same-sex couples. *Int J Palliat Nurs.* 2009;15(4):170–176.

35. Puchalski C, Ferrell B, Virani R, et al. Improving the quality of spiritual care as a dimension of palliative care: the report of the consensus conference. *J Palliat Med.* 2009;12(10):885–904.

36. Pulchalski C, Ferrell B. *Making Health Care Whole: Integrating Spirituality.* West Conshohocken, PA: Templeton Press; 2010.

37. Lynch S. Hospice and palliative care access issues in rural areas. *Am J Hospice Palliat Med.* 2012;30:172–177. doi:10.1177/1049909112444592.

38. Center to Advance Palliative Care; National Palliative Care Research Center. Report card: America's care of serious illness. A state-by-state report card on access to palliative care in our nation's hospitals. http://reportcard.capc.org/pdf/state-by-state-report-card.pdf. New York, NY: Center to Advance Palliative Care and National Palliative Care Research Center, 2011. Accessed April 3, 2015.

39. Madigan EA, Wiencek CA, Vander Schrier AL. Patterns of community-based end-of-life care in rural areas of the United States. *Policy Politics Nurs Pract.* 2009:10(1):71–81.

40. Heflt PR. To keep them from injustice: reflections on the care of unauthorized immigrants with cancer. *J Onc Pract.* 2012:8(4):212–214.

41. Dahlin CM. Communication in palliative care: An essential competency for nurses. In: Ferrell BR, Coyle N, eds. *Oxford Textbook of Palliative Nursing.* 4th ed. New York, NY: Oxford University Press; 2010:107–133.

42. Butow P, Bella M, Goldstein D, et al. Grappling with cultural differences; communication between oncologists and immigrant cancer patients with and without interpreters. *Patient Educ Couns.* 2011:84:398–405

43. Williams SW, Hanson LC, Boyd C, et al. Communication, decision making, and cancer: What African Americans want physicians to know. *J Palliat Med.* 2008;11:1221–1226.

44. Barclay JS, Blackhall LJ, Tulsky JA. Communication strategies and cultural issues in the delivery of bad news. *J Palliat Med.* 2007;10:958–977.

45. Foley H, Mazanec P. Culture and considerations in palliative care. In Panke JT, Coyne P, eds. *Conversations in Palliative Care.* 3rd ed. Pittsburgh, PA: Hospice & Palliative Nurses Association; 2011:157–163.

46. Patient Self-determination Act of 1990, 42 USC §§1395cc(a)(1)(Q), 1395cc(f).

47. Hsiung YY, Ferrans CE. Recognizing Chinese Americans' cultural needs in making end-of-life treatment decisions. *J Hosp Palliat Nurs.* 2007;9:132–140.

48. Taxis JC. Mexican Americans and hospice care: culture, control, and communication. *J Hosp Palliat Nurs.* 2008;10:133–161.

49. Schultz M, Bar-Sela G. Initiating palliative care conversations: lessons from Jewish bioethics. *J Support Onc.* 2013;11(1):1–7. (accessed June 20, 2013).

50. Artificial nutrition and hydration in end-of-life care [Hospice and Palliative Nurses Association position statement]. Pittsburgh, PA: Hospice and Palliative Nurses Association; June 2003. http://hpna.advancingexpertcare.

org/wp-content/uploads/2014/09/Artificial-Nutrition-and-Hydration-in-Advanced-Illness-FINAL.pdf. Accessed June 24, 2013.

51. McCaffery M, Pasero C. *Pain: Clinical Manual*. 2nd ed. St. Louis, MO: Mosby; 1999.

52. Wadner LD, Scipio CD, Hirsch AT, Torres CA, Robinson ME. The perception of pain in others: how gender, race and age influence pain expectations. *J Pain*. 2012;13:220–227. doi:10.1016/j.pain.2011.10.014.

53. Reynolds KS, Hanson LC, Henderson M, Steinhauser KE. End-of-life care in nursing home settings: do race or age matter? *Palliat Support Care*. 2008;6:21–27.

54. Gerdner LA, Yang D, Tripp-Reimer T. The circle of life: end-of-life care and death rituals for Hmong-American elders. *J Gerontol Nurs*. 2007;33:20–29.

55. O'Mallon MO. Vulnerable populations: exploring a family perspective of grief. *J Hospice Palliat Nurs*. 2009;11:91–98.

56. Campinha-Bacote J. A model and instrument for addressing cultural competence in health care. *J Nurs Educ*. 1999;38:203–207.

57. Hallarman L, Kearns C. The military history as a vehicle for exploring end-of-life care with veterans. *J Palliat Med*. 2008;11:104–105.

58. Bixby KA, Bateman J. Caring for veterans. In Panke JT, Coyne P, eds. *Conversations in Palliative Care*. 3rd ed. Pittsburgh, PA: Hospice and Palliative Nurses Association; 2011:283–294.

59. Nyatanga B. Cultural competence: a noble idea in a changing world. *Int J Palliat Nurs*. 2008;14:315.

Chapter 4

Meaning in Illness

Tami Borneman and Katherine Brown-Saltzman

Is it possible to adequately articulate and give definition to meaning in illness? Or is meaning in illness better described and understood through symbolism and metaphors? To try to define that which is enigmatic and bordering on the ineffable seems almost sacrilegious. The journey of finding meaning in illness, experienced by each patient facing the end of life and his or her family caregiver, would seem to be diminished by the process that seeks to understand through the use of language.

Is it that we seek to find meaning in illness, or is it that we seek to find meaning in the life now left and in relationships and things we value? Do we seek to find meaning in illness as an isolated event or that which is beyond the illness, such as how to live out this newly imposed way of life? Terminal illness often forces us to reappraise our life's meaning and purpose. If we allow space in our lives for the meaning in illness to unfold, we move from the superficial to the profound.

Terminal illness forces us to look directly at death, yet we resist the feelings that arise. Everything in us seeks and hopes for life. Everything in us denies death. There is something very cold, unmoving, and disturbing about it all. Does the end of one's human existence on Earth need to be the sole metaphor for death?

Although end of life issues are now nearer to the forefront of healthcare, the dying patient still faces an impersonal, detached, and cure-focused system. As necessary as it is for nurses to use the nursing process, it is not enough. The patient's illness beckons us to go beyond assessment, diagnosis, intervention, and evaluation to a place of vulnerability, not in an unprofessional manner but, rather, in a way that allows for a shared connectedness in each patient–nurse relationship. We need to be willing to use feelings appropriately as part of the therapeutic process. Separating ourselves from touching and feeling to protect ourselves only serves to make us more vulnerable, because we have placed our emotions in isolation. Nurses can help the patient and family find meaning in the illness and, in the process, help define or redefine their own meaning in life, illness, and death.

Meaning Defined

Johnston-Taylor[1] presents several definitions for *meaning* (Table 4.1). In the dictionary,[2] one finds *meaning* defined simply as "something that is conveyed

Table 4.1 Definitions of Meaning

Meaning	"refers to sense, or coherence.... A search for meaning implies a search for coherence. 'Purpose' refers to intention, aim, function.... however, 'purpose' of life and 'meaning' of life are used interchangeably."[4]
	"a structure which relates purposes to expectations so as to organise actions.... Meaning ... makes sense of actions by providing reasons for it."[5]
[Search for] meaning	"is an effort to understand the event: why it happened and what impact it has had ... [and] attempts to answer the question(s), What is the significance of the event?... What caused the event to happen? ... [and] What does my life mean now?"[6]
	"is an attempt to restore the sense that one's life was orderly and purposeful"[7]
Personal search for meaning	"the process by which a person seeks to interpret a life circumstance. The search involves questioning the personal significance of a life circumstance, in order to give the experience purpose and to place it in the context of a person's total life pattern. The basis of the process is the interaction between meaning in and of life and involves the reworking and redefining of past meaning while looking for meaning in a current life circumstance."[8]

or signified" or as "an interpreted goal, intent, or end." But it is the etymology of the word *mean* that helps nurses understand our potential for supporting patients in finding meaning in their lives, even as they face death. *Mean* comes from the Old English *maenan,* "to tell of." One does not find meaning in a vacuum; it has everything to do with relationships, spirituality, and connectedness. While the process of finding meaning depends greatly on an inward journey, it also relies on the telling of that journey. The telling may use language, but it may also be conveyed by the eyes, through the hands, or just in the way the body is held. Frankl[3] reminds us that the "will to meaning" is a basic drive for all of humanity and is unique to each individual. A life-threatening illness begs the question of meaning with a new urgency and necessity.

Cassell[9] tells us that "all events are assigned meaning," which entails judging their significance and value. Meaning cannot be separated from the person's past; it requires the thought of future and ultimately influences perception of that future (p. 67). Finding meaning is not a stagnant process; it changes as each day unfolds and the occurrences are interpreted. As one patient reflected upon his diagnosis, "Even though I have this I am still a whole person ... my thoughts are different, my ambitions are a little different because I want to spend as much time as I can with my grandkids."[10] Coming face to face with one's mortality not only defines what is important but also the poignancy of the loss of much that has been meaningful.

One's spirituality is often the key to transcending those losses and finding ways to maintain those connections, whether it is the belief that one's love, work, or creativity will remain after the physical separation, or that one's spirit goes on to an afterlife or through reincarnation. Meaning in life concerns the individual's realm of life on Earth. It has to do with one's humanness, the temporal, what one has done in life to give it meaning. The meaning of life has more to do with the existential, looking beyond one's earthly physical existence to an eternal, secure, and indelible God or spiritual plane. The existential realm of life provides a sense of security whereby one can integrate experiences.[11]

Spirituality has been defined as a search for meaning.[12,13] One of the Hebrew words for *meaning* is *biynah* (bee-naw), which is understanding, knowledge, and wisdom. It comes from the root word *biyn* (bene), to separate mentally or to distinguish.[14] How is it that one can come to knowledge and understanding? Patients receiving palliative care often describe a sense of isolation and loneliness. They frequently have endless hours available, while at the same time experiencing a shortening of their life. It is here that nurses have a pivotal role as listeners, for when the ruminations of the dying are given voice, there is an opportunity for meaning. Important life themes are shared, and the unanswerable questions are at least asked. As the stranger develops intimacy and trust, meaning takes hold.

Suffering creates one of the greatest challenges to uncovering meaning. For the dying patient, suffering comes in many packages: physical pain, unrelenting symptoms (nausea, pruritus, dyspnea, etc.), spiritual distress, dependency, multiple losses, and anticipatory grieving. Even the benefits of medical treatments given to provide hope or palliation can sometimes be outweighed by side effects (e.g., sedation and constipation from pain medication), inducing yet further suffering. The dictionary defines *suffering* in this way: "To feel pain or distress; sustain loss, injury, harm, or punishment."[2] But once again, it is the root word that allows for a more primitive understanding—the Latin *sufferre*, which comprises *sub,* "below," and *ferre,* "to carry." The weight and isolation of that suffering becomes more real at the visceral level. Cassell[9] reminds us that pain itself does not foreordain suffering; it is, in fact, the meaning that is attributed to that pain that determines the suffering. In his clinical definition, "[s]uffering is a state of severe distress induced by the loss of the intactness of person, or by a threat that the person believes will result in the loss of his or her intactness" (p. 63). Clinicians can further unnecessary suffering, as attested in the research of Berglund et al. by making patients feel objectified or by providing fragmented care.[15] Suffering is an individual and private experience, greatly influenced by the personality and character of the person; for example, the patient who has needed control during times of wellness will find the out-of-control experience of illness as suffering.[9] In writing about cancer pain and its meaning, Ersek and Ferrell[16] provide a summary of hypotheses and theses from the literature (Table 4.2).

Although not always recognized, it is the duty of all who care for patients to alleviate suffering, not just treat the illness's physical dimensions. This is no small task, as professionals must first be free from denial and the need to self-protect to see another's suffering. Then, they must be able to attend to it without trying to fix or simplify it. The suffering needs to be witnessed; in the midst of suffering, presence and compassion become the balm and hope for its relief.

Table 4.2 Summary of Hypotheses and Theses From the Literature on Meaning

Hypothesis/Thesis	Authors
The search for meaning is a basic human need.	Frankl 1959.[3]
Meaning is necessary for human fulfillment.	Steeves and Kahn 1987.[17]
Finding meaning fosters positive coping and increased hopefulness.	Ersek 1991[18]; Steeves and Kahn 1987[17]; Taylor 1983.[7]
One type of meaning-making activity in response to threatening events is to develop causal attributions.	Gotay 1983[19]; Haberman 1987[20]; Steeves and Kahn 1987[17]; Taylor 1983[7]; Chrisman and Haberman 1977.[21]
Meaning making can involve the search for a higher order.	Ersek 1991[18]; Ferrell et al. 1993[22]; Steeves and Kahn 1987.[17]
Making meaning often involves the use of social comparisons.	Ferrell et al. 1993[22]; Taylor 1983[7]; Ersek 1991[18]; Haberman 1987.[20]
Meaning can be derived through construing benefits from a negative experience.	Ersek 1991[18]; Haberman 1987[20]; Taylor 1983.[7]
Meaning sometimes focuses on illness as challenge, enemy, or punishment.	Barkwell 1991[23]; Ersek 1991[18]; Lipowski 1970.[24]
Pain and suffering often prompt a search for meaning.	Frankl 1959[3]; Steeves and Kahn 1987[17]; Taylor 1983.[7]
Uncontrolled pain or overwhelming suffering hinder the experience of meaning.	Steeves and Kahn 1987.[17]
One goal of care is to promote patients' and caregivers' search for and experiences of meaning.	Ersek 1991[18]; Ferrell et al. 1993[22]; Steeves and Kahn 1987[17]; Haberman 1988.[25]

The Process of Finding Meaning in Illness

From years of working with terminally ill patients and their families, the authors have found that the process of finding meaning in illness invokes many themes. The title given to each theme is an attempt to represent observed transitions that many terminally ill patients experience. Not all patients experience the transitions in order, and not all transitions are experienced. However, we have observed that these transitions are experienced by the majority of patients. The themes shared in this section are the imposed transition, loss and confusion, the dark night of the soul, randomness and absence of God, brokenness, and reappraisal. In experiencing some or all of these transitions, one can perhaps find meaning in this difficult time of life.

The Imposed Transition

Being told that you have a terminal illness can be like hearing the sound of prison doors slam shut. Life will never be the same. The sentence has been handed down, and the verdict cannot be reversed. Terminal illness is a loss; there is nothing we can do to change the prognosis, even though we may temporarily delay the final outcome. The essence of our being is shaken, and our souls are stricken with a panic unlike any other we have ever felt. For the first time, we are faced with an "existential awareness of nonbeing."[26] For a brief moment, the silence is deafening, as if suspended between two worlds, the known and the unknown. As one "regains consciousness," the pain and pandemonium of thoughts and emotions begin to storm the floodgates of our faith, our coping abilities, and our internal fortitude. The word *terminal* reverberates in our heads. There is no easy or quick transition to terminal diagnosis acceptance.

Facing the end of life provokes self-reflective questions, including both the meaning *of* life and the meaning *in* life. Whether we embrace with greater fervor the people and things that collectively give us meaning in life or we view it all as now lost, the loss and pain are real. Nothing can prevent the inevitable. There is a sense of separation or disconnectedness: While I am the same person, I have become permanently different from you. Unless you become like me, diagnosed with a terminal illness, we are, in this sense, separated. In a rhetorical sense, the meanings we gain in life from relationships and the material world serve to affirm us as participants in these meanings.[26] When a terminal diagnosis threatens these meanings, we fear the loss of who we are as functioning, productive human beings. The affirmations we received from our meanings in life are now at a standstill.

A 65-year-old retired military man, although accepting of his prognosis, fought to delay the inevitable for as long as possible. As a military man, he was not afraid of dying. His relationship with one of his grown children was very good and he adored his grandchildren. They were the reason he was fighting the cancer. He felt that life was most enjoyable when he spent time with them. His concern about dying was that because the grandchildren were young, he would not have enough time for them to remember him after he died. "My grandkids are more important, you know, so 'course they got to remember their grandpa. I want them to think about me, what grandparents did you know?"[27] When we discussed how he might leave a legacy, he recognized that he saw himself and his remaining time in limited ways. He feared losing what had come to define his life. Encouraging him to redefine his life through leaving a legacy for his grandchildren gave him new insights and provided a practical way to spend his remaining time.

In addition to questioning meaning *in* life, those facing the end of life also question the meaning *of* life. A life-threatening illness makes it difficult to maintain an illusion of immortality.[28] What happens when we die? Is there really a God? Is it too late for reconciliation? For those believing in life after death, the questions may concern the uncertainty of eternal life, fear of what eternal life will be like, or the possibility of this being a test of faith. No matter which belief system, the end of life patient asks the existential questions. We reach out for a connection with God or something beyond one's self for security and stability. Then, in this ability to transcend the situation, ironically we somehow feel a sense of groundedness. Frankl[3] states, "It denotes the fact that being human always points, and is directed, to something or someone, other than oneself—be it a meaning to fulfill or another human being to encounter." There is an incredibly strong spiritual need to find meaning in this senseless and chaotic new world.

Loss and Confusion

One cancer patient stated, "Our lives are like big run-on sentences and when cancer occurs, it's like a period was placed at the end of the sentence. In reality, we all have a period at the end of the sentence, but we don't really pay attention to it."[29] With a terminal diagnosis, life is changed forever, for however long that life may be. Each day life changes, as one is forced to experience a new aspect of the loss. There is a sense of immortality that pervades our lust for life, and when we are made to look at our mortality, it is staggering. With the many losses, coupled with the fear of dying, one can be left confused by the infinite possibilities of the unknown. The panorama of suffering seems to be limitless.

The pain of loss is as great as the pleasure we derived from life.[30] The pain is pure and somewhat holy. The confusion comes not only from having one's world turned upside down, but also from those who love and care about us. It is not intentional; nevertheless, its impact is greatly felt. In trying to encourage or help us to find meaning, those around us may minimize the loss and pain by comparing losses, attempting to save God's reputation by denying the freedom to be angry at God, or by focusing on the time left to live. The hurting soul needs to feel the depth of the loss by whatever means it can. The pain from loss is relentless, like waves from a dark storm at sea, crashing repeatedly against rocks on the shoreline.

A 55-year-old woman with terminal lung cancer experienced further physical decline each day. She was supported by a husband who lovingly doted on her. She loved life and her family. She experienced many losses because of her comorbid conditions, along with the cancer. Her family's desire that she focus on life, and not on her disease or death, added to these losses. Her husband stated they were aware she was going to die, but felt that her quality of life would be better if these issues were not discussed. The patient had many thoughts and feelings to sort through; she wanted to talk, but no one was listening. Her loss was not just physical; it was also emotional, caused by a loving family trying to do the right thing. Many times the patient ended up in tearful frustration. Her family communications were different, a constant reminder that nothing was the same and, in turn, a reminder of her losses and impending death.

Captured in Tolstoy's *The Death of Ivan Ilyich*, we hear the agony of Ivan's similar experience: "This deception tortured him— their not wishing to admit what they all knew and what he knew, but wanting to lie to him concerning his terrible condition, and wishing and forcing him to participate in that lie. . . . And strangely enough, many times when they were going through their antics over him he had been within a hairbreadth of calling out to them: 'Stop lying! You know and I know that I am dying. Then at least stop lying about it!' But he had never had the spirit to do it."[31]

Dark Night of the Soul

The descent of darkness pervades every crack and crevice of one's being. One now exists in the place of Nowhere, surrounded by nothingness, devoid of texture and contour. One's signature is seemingly wiped away, taking with it the identification of a living soul.[30] Job states, "And now my soul is poured out within me; days of affliction have seized me. At night it pierces my bones within me, and my gnawing pains take no rest . . . My days are swifter than a weaver's shuttle, and come to an end without hope."[32] As Jerry Sittser writes, "One enters the abyss of emptiness—with the perverse twist that one is not empty of the tortured feeling of emptiness."[33] This is pain's infinite desert.

Darkness looms as one thinks about the past, full of people and things that provided meaning in life, things that will soon be given up. Darkness looms as one thinks about the future, because death precludes holding on to all that is loved and valued. Darkness consumes one's mind and heart, like fire consumes wood. It makes its way to the center with great fury, where it proceeds to take possession, leaving nothing but a smoldering heap of ashes and no hope of recovering any essence of life.[34]

A woman with fairly young children relapsed, after several years free of colon cancer. She received several months of treatment with an experimental protocol. She suffered greatly, not only from the effects of the chemotherapy, but also from the long periods of time not being able to "be there" for her children. When it became clear that the chemo was not working as expected, she became tortured by the thought of abandoning her children at a time when they so greatly needed a mother, and the fact that she had gambled with the little time she had left and had lost. Now in her mind, her children had the double loss of months of quality time she could have had with them and her impending death. She became inconsolable because of this darkness. Time to intervene was very limited. Allowing her the room for suffering, and being "present" to this suffering as a nurse, was essential. In addition, moving back into her mothering role and providing for her children by helping to prepare them for her death became the pathway through the darkness and into meaning.

Although one might try, there are no answers—theological or otherwise—to the "whys" that engulf one's existence. Death moves from an "existential phenomenon to a personal reality."[35] All our presuppositions about life fall away and we are left emotionally naked. There is no physical, emotional, or spiritual strength to help our fragility. The world becomes too big for us and our inner worlds are overwhelming.[30] The enigma of facing death strips order from one's life, creating fragmentation and leaving one with the awareness that life is no longer tenable.

Randomness and the Absence of God

The pronouncement of a terminal diagnosis provokes inner turmoil and ruminating thoughts from dawn to dusk. Even in one's chaotic life, there was order. But order does not always prevail. A young athlete being recruited for a professional sport is suddenly killed in a tragic car accident. A mother of three small children is diagnosed with a chronic debilitating disease that will end in death. An earthquake levels a brand new home for which a husband and wife had spent years saving. A playful young toddler drowns in a pool. There seems to be no reason. It would be different if negligence were involved. If the young athlete were speeding or driving drunk, although the loss still would be quite devastating, a "logical" reason could be assigned to it. But randomness leaves us with no "logical" explanation.[33]

The word *random* comes from the Middle English word *radon,* which is derived from the Old French word *randon,* meaning violence and speed. The word connotes an impetuous and haphazard movement, lacking careful choice, aim, or purpose.[2] The feeling of vulnerability is overwhelming. In an effort to find shelter from this randomness, we seek meaning and comfort from God or something beyond ourselves, but how do we know that God or something beyond ourselves is not the cause of our loss? Our trust is shaken. Can we reconcile God's sovereignty with our loss?[33] Can we stay connected to or gain strength and security from something that may be the originator of our pain? There is a sense of abandonment by that which has been our stronghold in life. Yet to cut ourselves off from that stronghold out of anger would leave us in a state of total disconnection. A sense of connection is a vital emotion necessary for existence, no matter how short that existence may be. But facing death forbids us to keep our existential questions and desires at a distance. Rather, it seems to propel us into a deeper search for meaning, as the questions continue to echo in our minds.

Brokenness

Does one come to a place of acceptance within brokenness? Is acceptance even attainable? Sometimes, sometimes not. Coming to a place of acceptance is an individual experience for each person. In a wonderful analogy of acceptance, Kearney[36] states, "Acceptance is not something an individual can choose at will. It is not like some light switch that can at will be flicked on or off. Deep emotional acceptance is like the settling of a cloud of silt in a troubled pool. With time the silt rests on the bottom and the water is clear" (p. 98). Brokenness does, however, open the door to relinquishing the illusion of immortality. Brokenness allows the soul to cry and to shed tears of anguish. It elicits the existential question "Why?" once again, only this time, not to gain answers, but to find meaning.

A woman in her mid-60s, dying of lung cancer, shared how she came to a place of acceptance. When she was first diagnosed, the cancer was already well advanced. Her health rapidly declined, and she was more or less confined to bed or sitting. Out of her frustration, anger at God, sadness, and tears came the desire to paint again. It was her way of coping, but it became more than that. It brought her to a place of peace in her heart. She had gotten away from painting because of busyness and was now learning to be blessed by quietness. She was very good at creating cards with her own designs, in watercolor, leaving the insides blank to be filled in by the giver. She would give these cards away to many people as her gesture of love and gratitude.

A gradual perception occurs, whereby we realize that the way out is by no longer struggling.[36] When we come to the end of ourselves and the need to fight the inevitable that is death, we give space for meaning to unfold. It is not that we give up the desire, but we relinquish the need to emotionally turn the situation around and to have all our questions answered. Sittser,[33] a minister who experienced a sudden loss of several immediate family members, states, "My experience taught me that loss reduces people to a state of almost total brokenness and vulnerability. I did not simply feel raw pain; I was raw pain" (p. 164). Pain and loss are still profound, but in the midst of these heavy emotions, there begins to be a glimmer of light. Like the flame of a candle, the light may wax and wane. It is enough to begin to silhouette those people and things that still can provide meaning.

Reappraisal

It is here one begins to realize that something positive can come from even a terminal diagnosis and the losses it imposes. The good that is gained does not mitigate the pain of loss but, rather, fosters hope—hope that is not contingent on healing but on reconciliation, on creating memories with loved ones, on making the most of every day, on loving and being loved.[37] It is a hope that transcends science and explanations and changes with the situation. It is not based on a particular outcome but, rather, focuses on the future, however long that may be. Despair undermines hope, but hope robs death of despair.[38]

A male patient in his late 30s, facing the end of life after battling leukemia and having gone through a bone marrow transplant, shared that he knew he was going to die. It took him a long time to be able to admit it to himself. The patient recalled recently visiting a young man who had basically given up and did not want his last dose of chemotherapy. He talked awhile with this young man and encouraged him to "go for it." He told him that there is nothing like watching the last drop of chemo go down the tube and into his body, and the sense of it finally being all over. The patient shared with the young man that when he received his own last dose of chemotherapy, he stayed up until three in the morning to watch the last drop go down the tube. Although the chemotherapy did not help him to the extent that he wanted, he wanted to encourage the young man to hope and not give up. Life was not yet over. He had tears in his eyes when he finished the story.

Facing end of life with a terminal diagnosis will never be a happy event. It will always be tragic, because it causes pain and loss to everyone involved. But at a time unique to each person facing death, a choice can be made as to whether one wants to become bitter and devalue the remaining time, or to value the time that is left as much as possible.

An important choice during this time is whether to forgive or to be unforgiving—toward oneself, others, God, or one's stronghold of security in life. Being unforgiving breeds bitterness and superficiality. As we face the end of life, we need both an existential connection and a connection with others. Being unforgiving separates us from those connections, and it is only through forgiveness that the breach is healed. Forgiveness neither condones another's actions, nor does it mean that this terminal diagnosis is fair. Rather, forgiveness is letting go of expectations that one somehow will be vindicated for the pain and loss. Whether by overt anger or by emotional withdrawal, in seeking to avoid vulnerability to further pain and loss, we only succeed in making ourselves more vulnerable. Now we have chosen a deeper separation that goes beyond facing the death of the physical body—that of the soul.[33] Positive vulnerability through forgiveness provides a means of healing and, when possible, reconciliation with others. It always provides healing and reconciliation with one's God or one's stronghold of security. Forgiveness allows both physical and emotional energy to be used for creating and enjoying the time left for living.

A 30-year-old woman was admitted to the hospital with advanced metastatic breast cancer. She was unknown to the hospital staff but had a good relationship with her oncologist. During the admissions assessment, the young woman could not give the name of anyone to contact in the event of an emergency. When pressed, she stated that she was alienated from her family and chose not to be in touch. She agreed that after her death her mother could be called, but not before. A social worker was summoned in the hope that something could be done to help with some unification. However, the social worker came out of the room devastated by the woman's resolve. The chaplain also found no way to reconnect this woman's family. The nursing staff experienced moral distress as they watched this woman die, all alone in the world. One of the authors worked with the staff to help them realize that they had become trusted, and in a sense were her substitute family. One may not always be able to fix the pain of life's fractures or bring people to a place of forgiveness, but it is important not to underestimate what is happening in the moment. Healing for this patient came through the relationship with her doctors and nurses, and she died not alone, but cared for.

There are many emotions and issues with which those facing death must contend. It is not an easy journey and the process is wearing; nevertheless, the rose can be found.

Impact of the Terminal Illness on the Patient–Caregiver Relationship

Each of us comes to new situations with our life's experiences and the meanings we have gained from them. It is no different when being confronted with illness and the end of life. However, in this special episode of life, there are often no personal "reruns" from which to glean insight. Patient and family come together as novices, each helping the other through this unknown passage. Because different roles and relationships exist, the impending loss will create different meanings for each person involved.

Facing the loss of someone you love is extremely difficult. For the family caregiver, the process of finding meaning is influenced by the one facing death. One example experienced by one of the authors involved a wife's discussion with her terminally ill husband over several months regarding his outlook on life. As Christians, they knew where death would take them, but she was curious as to what that meant to him and how he was handling the unknown. She felt strong in her own faith, but also felt like she was giving lip service to it at times. He described life as having even more meaning; although he loved her and the life they had together very much, he could now "cherish" every moment of that time. He was sad knowing that he would eventually die from the cancer, but until that time came, he just wanted to enjoy life with her. She shared that while what he said seemed obvious when he said it, for some reason this time, it really spoke to her soul and she felt peace.

In another example, a woman helped her family create meaning from the picture she had painted of herself sitting on the beach as a little girl next to a little boy. She explained that the little boy had his arm around her as they stared out at the sea. Each time the waves covered the surface of the beach and then retreated, the sea would carry with it bits and pieces of her fears and disease. The birds circling overhead would then swoop down to pick up and carry off any pieces not taken by the sea. The little boy's arm around her signified all the loving support she had received from others. When the time came for her to die, she would be ready, because she had been able to let go of life as she knew it. She had let the waves slowly carry that which was of life out to sea, yet she had learned to hold on to the meaning that that life had represented. In doing so, she enabled her family to hold on to the meaning of their relationship with her, and to remain symbolically connected after her death.

A poignant final story offers a different perspective. A 60-year-old woman with stage IV ovarian cancer was very angry at her husband and perplexed at God. She had trouble finding any positive meaning in anything in life. She was upset that her life would be cut short, and she never had children. She blamed her husband for not wanting to have children, after the surgeon told her that never having children increased the risk for ovarian cancer. She resented the fact that she had lived in a difficult marriage and now "this" was happening to her. She felt horrible for having these feelings, because she didn't like feeling this way. She also dealt with an obsessive-compulsive disorder (OCD) regarding cleanliness that made life miserable for herself and those around her. This presented problems for the family in trying to care for her because as the cancer got worse, she needed more physical care, but the OCD presented a barrier not easily maneuvered around, leaving family members exhausted and frustrated. The family felt like they could give her much better care, but were prevented from doing so. This was extremely difficult for them. When the patient died, their relationships were very good, but the family had spent a lot of time talking about what all of this meant to them. They were able to talk about the positives and negatives and realized that they did the best they could, given the patient-imposed limitations.

We present these actual patient stories to exemplify how the patient's meaning in illness affects the meaning held or created by family members. Differing or divergent meanings can be detrimental in a relationship, or can be used to strengthen it, thereby increasing the quality of time left together. That is not to imply that the patient is responsible for the meaning created by family members; rather, they are responsible for how one affects the other. Germino, Fife, and Funk[39] suggest that the goal is not merely converging meanings within the patient–family dyad but, rather, encouraging a sharing of individual meanings so that all can learn, and relationships can be deepened and strengthened.

Family caregivers face many issues in caring for a loved one nearing the end of life. They are discussed at length in the literature. There is one issue, however, that warrants more attention: the loss of dreams, and with it the loss of dreams for a future with the person. It is the loss of the way one used to imagine life and how it would have been with that person. It is the loss of an emotional image of oneself and the abandonment of chosen plans for the future and what might have been.[40]

For a child and the surviving parent, those losses of dreams will be played out each time Mother's or Father's Day arrives and at important life-cycle events, such as graduations, weddings, or the birth of the first grandchild. As her mother lay dying, one child expressed that loss in the simple statement, "Mommy, you won't be here for my birthday!" The mother and child wept, holding and comforting each other. Nothing could change the loss, but the comforting would remain forever.

The loss of dreams is an internal process, spiritual for some, and seldom recognized by others as needing processing.[29,40-42] At this point, nurses have a wonderful opportunity to verbally recognize the family caregivers' loss of dreams and to encourage them in their search to find meaning in the loss. The ability to transcend and connect to God, or something greater than one's self, helps the healing process.

Transcendence: Strength for the Journey That Lies Ahead

Transcendence is defined as lying beyond the ordinary range of perception; being above and independent of the material universe. The Latin root is trans-, "from or beyond," plus scandere, "to climb."[2] The images are many: the man in a pit climbing his way out one handhold at a time; the story of Job as he endured one defeat after another and yet found meaning; the climber who reaches the mountaintop, becoming closer to the heavens while still having the connection to the earth; or the dying patient who, in peace, is already seeing into another reality. The ability to transcend truly is a gift of the human spirit and often comes after a long struggle and bout of suffering. It is often unclear which comes first—does meaning open the door for transcendence, or, quite the opposite, does the act of transcendence bring the meaning? More than likely, it is an intimate dance between the two, one fueling the other. In the Buddhist tradition, suffering and being are a totality, and integrating suffering in this light becomes an act of transcendence.[43]

Transcendence of suffering can also be accomplished by viewing it as reparation for sins while still living—preparing the way for eternity, as in the Islamic tradition. In other traditions, transcendence is often relationship-based, the connection to others, and sometimes to a higher power.[3] For example, the

Christian seeing Christ on the cross is connected to the relationship and endurance of God and the reality that suffering is a part of life. For others, it is finding meaning in relating to others, even the act of caring for others. And for some, that relationship may be with the Earth, a sense of stewardship and leaving the environment a better place. It is rare that patients reach a state of transcendence and remain there through their dying. Instead, for most, it is a process in which there are moments when they reach a sense of expansion that supports them in facing death. The existential crisis does not rule, because one can frame the relationship beyond death; for example, "I will remain in their hearts and memories forever, I will live on through my children, or my spirit will live beyond my limited physical state."

Nursing Interventions

If one returns to the root word of meaning, *maenan,* or "to tell of," this concept can be the guide that directs the nurse toward interventions. Given the nature of this work, interventions may not be the true representation of what is needed. For intervention implies action, that the nurse has an answer and she can direct the course of care by intervening. It is defined as "[t]o come, appear, or lie between two things. To come in or between so as to hinder or alter an action."[2] But finding meaning is process-oriented; while finely honed psychosocial skills and knowledge can be immensely helpful, there is no bag of tricks. One example would be of a chaplain who walks into the room and relies only on offering prayer to the patient, preventing any real discourse or relationship-building. The patient's personhood has been diminished, and potentially, more harm than good has been done.

So let us revisit "to tell of." What is required of the professional who enters into the healing dimension of a patient's suffering and search for meaning? It would seem that respect may be the starting point—respect for that individual's way of experiencing suffering and his or her attempts at making sense of the illness. Second, allow for an environment and time for the telling. Even as this is written, the sighs of frustration are heard: "We have no time!" If nursing fails at this, if nurses turn their backs on their intrinsic promise to alleviate suffering, then nursing can no longer exist. Instead, the nurse becomes, simply, the technician and the scheduler—the nurse becomes a part of the problem. She has violated the ANA Code of Ethics for Nurses that asserts nurses are obligated to address the alleviation of suffering and provide supportive care to the dying: "The measures nurses take to care for the patient enable the patient to live with as much physical, emotional, social, and spiritual well-being as possible. This is particularly vital in the care of patients and their families at the end of life to prevent and relieve the cascade of symptoms and suffering that are commonly associated with dying."[44]

If patients in the midst of suffering receive the message, nonverbally or directly, that there is no time, energy, or compassion, they will, in their vulnerability, withdraw or become needier. When patients feel distrusted, objectified, and overlooked, they suffer at the hands of those who were to provide care.[15] Their alienation becomes complete. On the other hand, if privacy and a moment of honor and focused attention are provided, this allows for the tears to spill or the anguish to be spoken. Then the alienation is broken, and the opportunity for healing one dimension is begun. The terminally ill are a vulnerable population. They die and do not complete patient satisfaction surveys; their grievances and their stories die with them. But the violation does not, for each nurse now holds that violation, as does society as a whole. The wound begets wounds, and the nurse sinks further into the protected and unavailable approach, alienated. The work holds no rewards, only endless days and demands. She or he has nothing left to give. The patient and family are ultimately abandoned. In the work of Kahn and Steeves,[45] one finds a model for the nurse's role in psychosocial processes and suffering. It represents the dynamic relationship of caring, acted out in caregiving as well as in the patient's coping, which transform each other.

For the nurse to provide this level of caregiving, he or she must understand the obstructions that may interfere. It is essential that the nurse undergo his or her own journey, visiting the intense emotions around the dying process and the act of witnessing suffering. We can serve the suffering person best if we ourselves are willing to be transformed through the process of our own grief as well as by the grief of others.[46] Presence may, in fact, be our greatest gift to these patients and their families. Still, imagine charting or accounting for presence on an acuity system! Presence "transcends role obligations and acknowledges the vulnerable humanness of us all . . . to be present means to unconceal, to be aware of tone of voice, eye contact, affect, and body language, to be in tune with the patient's messages."[46] Presence provides confirmation, nurturing, and compassion and is an essential transcendent act.

Touch becomes one of the tools of presence and is valued by the dying and their families.[47,48] Used with sensitivity, it can be as simple as the holding of the hand or as powerful as the holding of the whole person. Sometimes, because of agitation or pain, direct touch becomes intrusive; even then, touch can be invoked, by the touching of a pillow or the sheet or the offering of a cold cloth. Healing touch takes on another level of intention through the directing energy of prayer.

If a key aspect of meaning is to tell, then one might be led to believe that the spoken word would be imperative. However, over and over, it is silence that conveys the meaning of suffering, "a primitive form of existence that is without an effective voice and imprisoned in silence." Compassionate listeners in respect and presence become mute themselves.[46] They use the most intuitive skills to carry the message. This may also be why other approaches that use symbols, metaphors, and the arts are the most potent in helping the patient to communicate and make sense of meaning. The arts, whether writing, music, or visual arts, often help the patient not only gain new insight, but convey that meaning to others. There are many levels on which this is accomplished. Whether it is done passively, through reading poetry, listening to music, or viewing paintings, or actively through creation, thoughts can be inspired, feelings moved, and the sense of connectedness and being understood can evolve. What once was ubiquitous can now be seen outside of one's soul, as feelings become tangible. It can be relational, because the act of creation can link one to the creator, or it can downplay the role of dependency, as the ill one now cares for others with a legacy of creational gifts.[49]

Meditation and or yoga are other acts of transcendence that can be extremely powerful for the dying.[50-53] Even those who have never experienced a meditational state can find that this new world, in many ways, links them to living and dying. The relaxation response from meditation or yoga allows the anxious patient to escape into a meditative state, experiencing an element of control while relinquishing control. Many patients describe it as a floating state, a time of great peace and calm. Some who have never had such an experience can find the first time frightening, as the existential crisis, quelled so well by boundaries, is no longer confined. Most, given a trusting and safe teacher, will find that meditation will serve them well. The meditation can be in the form of prayer, guided imagery, breathing techniques, or mantras.

Prayer is well documented in the literature[54-56] as having meaning for patients and families; not only does it connect one to God, but it also again becomes a relational connection to others. Knowing that one is prayed for not only by those close at hand but by strangers, communities, and those at a great distance can be deeply nurturing. Often forgotten is the role in which the patient can be empowered, that of praying for others. One of the authors experienced her patient's prayers for her; the tables were turned, and the patient became the healer. The patient suddenly lost the sense of worthlessness and glowed with joy.

Leaving a legacy may be one of the most concrete ways for patients to find meaning in this last stage of their lives.[57] It most often requires the mastering of the existential challenges, in which patients know that death is at hand and choose to direct their course and what they leave behind. For some patients, that will mean going out as warriors, fighting until the end; for others, it will mean end of life planning that focuses on quality of life. Some patients will design their funerals, using rituals and readings that reveal their values and messages for others. Others will create videos, write letters, or distribute their wealth in meaningful ways. Blogging is a way to decrease a sense of isolation for patients, as they record their experiences and also leave a permanent imprint of their lives on the Internet.[58] It becomes a diary of the illness that has been shown to increase a sense of purpose and meaning as patients share with others.[58,59] Parents who are leaving young children sometimes have the greatest difficulty with this aspect. On one hand, the feelings of horror at "abandoning" their children are so strong that they have great difficulty facing their death. Still, there is often a part of them that has this need to leave a legacy. The tug-of-war between these two willful emotions tends to leave only short windows of opportunity to prepare. The extreme can be observed in the young father who began to push his toddler away, using excuses for the distancing. It was only after a trusting relationship had been established with one of the authors that she could help him to see how this protective maneuver was, in fact, harming the child. The father not only needed to see what he was doing, but to see how his love would help the child and how others would be there for the child and wife in their pain and grief. With relief, the father reconnected with his young son, creating living memories and a lifetime protection of love.

Another courageous parent, anticipating the missed birthdays, bought cards and wrote a note in each one, so that the child would be touched not only by the individual messages, but the knowledge that the parent found a way to be there for him on each year. A mother wrote a note for her young daughter, so that if she should ever marry, she would have a gift to be opened on her wedding day. The note described the mother's love, wisdom about marriage, and her daughter's specialness, already known through a mother's eyes. An elderly person may write or tape an autobiography or even record the family tree, lest it be lost with the passing of a generation. The nurse can often inspire these acts, but he or she must always do so with great care, so as not to instill a sense of "should" or "must," which would add yet another burden.

Helping patients to reframe hope is another important intervention.[60] Dr. William Breitbart, chief of psychiatry services at Memorial Sloan Kettering Cancer Center in New York City, designed and conducted research on a meaning-centered psychotherapeutic intervention to help terminally ill patients with cancer maintain hope and meaning as they face the end of their lives.[4] This research was inspired by the works of Dr. Victor Frankl, a psychiatrist and Holocaust survivor. Cancer patients attended an 8-week, group-focused, standardized course of experiential exercises that addressed constructs of despair at the end of life, such as hopelessness, depression, loss of meaning, suicidal ideation, and desire for a hastened death. The study revealed that the patient's spiritual well-being, specifically the loss of meaning, was more highly correlated to the components that made up despair at the end of life than either depression or hopelessness alone. As a result, if the patient could manipulate or reframe his/her sense of meaning and spiritual well-being, this would positively affect the foundational elements of despair at the end of life. When patients are able to do this, they are able to sustain their hope, because they have been able to reframe the focus of their hope.

The Healthcare Professional

Although the healthcare professional can be educated about death and grieving, like the patient and family, it is in the professional's living out the experience that he or she reaches an understanding. It is a developmental process, and given the demands of the work, the nurse is at great risk for turning away from her feelings. Often little mentoring accompanies a nurse's first deaths, let alone formal debriefing or counseling. How can it be that we leave such important learning to chance? And what about cumulative losses and the years of witnessing suffering? Healthcare needs to include healing rituals, for all of its healthcare professionals, to support and guide them in this work. Individual institutions can develop programs that address these needs.

At one institution, "Teas for the Soul" (sponsored by the Pastoral Care Department) provides respite in the workplace on a regular basis and after difficult deaths or traumas. A cart with cookies and tea, as well as soft music, are provided to nurture the staff physically and emotionally and to come together in support. A renewal program, the "Circle of Caring," is a retreat that supports healthcare professionals from a variety of institutions in a weekend of self-care that integrates spirituality, the arts, and community building. The element of suffering is a focal point for a small-group process that addresses the effects of the work and teaches skills and rituals for coping with its ongoing demands.

Perhaps one of the most challenging aspects of a nurses's finding meaning is when he or she sees nonbeneficial treatment continued and palliative care is forestalled. The nurse experiences not only the normal emotional burden of caring for the dying, but now has the added weight and guilt of feeling that she or he is contributing to harming the patient. While healthcare professionals need to address the nonbeneficial treatment and refocus on appropriate goals of care in the interim, nurses and the entire healthcare team need to attend to the moral distress. Research has demonstrated that speaking up clearly makes a lasting impact on moral distress and yet, often, the moral distress is not addressed. Failure to do so may result in the crescendo effect, detaching from patients, or even leaving the profession.[61-63] Ultimately, even if constrained by a lack of DNR orders or continued burdensome treatments, the nurse can focus her or his intentions on what she/he is able to do for the patient and family. Whether it is treating the patient with respect and tenderness or humanizing the experience through the simplest of acts (offering music, the reading of a poem, or comfort to those at the bedside), an awareness of the moral action of caring, so essential to nursing, will not only improve the care but the nurse's resiliency.

Clearly, there is much that can be done to support nurses individually and to support organizations. There are many opportunities for assisting nurses in their own search for meaning and for enhancing the care of patients and families. When the nurse takes the time to find meaning in this work, she or he finds a restorative practice that will protect him or her personally and professionally. Like the patient, she or he will need to choose this journey and find pathways that foster, challenge, and renew.

> *As long as we can love each other,*
> *And remember the feeling of love we had,*
> *We can die without ever really going away.*
> *All the love you created is still there.*
> *All the memories are still there.*
> *You live on—in the hearts of everyone you have*
> *Touched and nurtured while you were here.*
> *—Morrie Schwartz*[64]

References

1. Taylor EJ. Whys and wherefores: adult patient perspectives of the meaning of cancer. *Semin Oncol Nurs.* 1995;11(1):32–40.

2. *The American Heritage Dictionary of the English Language.* Houghton Mifflin; 2013.

3. Frankl VE. *Man's Search for Meaning: An Introduction to Logotherapy.* Boston: Beacon; 1959.

4. Breitbart W. Reframing hope: meaning-centered care for patients near the end of life. Interview by Karen S. Heller. *J Palliat Med.* 2003;6(6):979–988.

5. Yalom ID. *Existential Psychotherapy*. New York, NY: Basic Books; 1980.

6. Marris P. *Loss and Change*. 2nd ed. London: Routledge and Kegan Paul; 1986.

7. Taylor SE. Adjustment to threatening events: A theory of cognitive adaptation. *Am Psychology*. 1983;38:1161–1173.

8. O'Connor AP, Wicker CA, Germino BB. Understanding the cancer patient's search for meaning. *Cancer Nurs*. 1990;13(3):167–175.

9. Cassell EJ: The relationship between pain and suffering. *Adv Pain Res Ther*. 1989;11:61–70.

10. Personal interview, 2007.

11. Koestenbaum P. *Is There an Answer to Death?* Englewood Cliffs, NJ: Prentice-Hall; 1976.

12. Puchalski C. Spirituality. In: Berger A, Shuster J, Roenn JV, eds. *Principles and Practice of Palliative Care and Supportive Oncology*. Philadelphia, PA: Lippincott Williams & Wilkins; 2013:702–718.

13. Vachon ML. Meaning, spirituality, and wellness in cancer survivors. *Semin Oncol Nurs*. 2008;24(3):218–225.

14. Strong's Exhaustive Concordance. 2013. Accessed June 27, 2013. http://www.biblestudytools.com/concordances/strongs-exhaustive-concordance/

15. Berglund M, Westin L, Svanstrom R, Sundler A. Suffering caused by care—patients' experiences from hospital settings. *Int J Qualitative Stud Health Well-being*. 2012;7:1–9.

16. Ersek M, Ferrell BR. Providing relief from cancer pain by assisting in the search for meaning. *J Palliat Care*. 1994;10(4):15–22.

17. Steeves RH, Kahn DL. Experience of meaning in suffering. *Image: J Nurs Scholarship*. 1987;19(3):114–116.

18. Ersek M. *The process of maintaining hope in adults with leukemia undergoing bone marrow transplantation* [unpublished doctoral dissertation]. Seattle: University of Washington; 1991.

19. Gotay CC. Why me? Attributions and adjustment by cancer patients and their mates at two stages in the disease process. *Soc Sci Med*. 1985;20(8):825–831.

20. Haberman MR. *Living with leukemia: The personal meaning attributed to illness and treatment by adults undergoing bone marrow transplantation* [unpublished doctoral dissertation]. Seattle; University of Washington; 1987.

21. Chrisman H. The health seeking process: an approach to the natural history of illness. *Culture, Med Psychiatry*. 1977;1(4):351–377.

22. Ferrell BR, Taylor EJ, Sattler GR, Fowler M, Cheyney BL. Searching for the meaning of pain: cancer patients', caregivers', and nurses' perspectives. *Cancer Pract*. 1993;1(3):185–194.

23. Barkwell DP. Ascribing meaning: A critical factor in coping and pain attenuation in patients with cancer-related pain. *J Palliat Care*. 1991;7(3):5–10.

24. Lipowski Z. Physical illness, the individual and their coping processes. *Int J Psychiatr Med*. 1970;1(9):101.

25. Haberman MR. Psychosocial aspects of bone marrow transplantation. *Semin Oncol Nurs*. 1988;4(1):55–59.

26. Tillich P. *The Courage to Be*. New Haven, CT: Yale University Press; 1952.

27. Personal interview, 1997.

28. Benson H. *Timeless Healing*. New York, NY: Simon & Schuster; 1997.

29. Putnam C. Personal communication. 1999.

30. O'Donohue J. *Eternal Echoes*. New York, NY: HarperCollins; 1999.

31. Tolstoy L. *The Death of Ivan Ilyich*. Maude L, Maude A, trans. Christian Classics Ethereal Library; originally published 1886. http://www.ccel.org/ccel/tolstoy/ivan.txt. Accessed November 1, 2013.

32. Job 30:16–17, 7:6. *New American Standard Bible*. Grand Rapids, MI: World Publishing; 1995.

33. Sittser JL. *A Grace Disguised: How the Soul Grows Through Loss*. Grand Rapids, MI: Zondervan Publishing, 1995.

34. St. John of the Cross. *Dark Night of the Soul*. Kila, MT: Kessinger Publishing, 2007; originally published 1542.

35. Kritek P. *Reflections on Healing*. Boston, MA: Jones & Bartlett; 2003.

36. Kearney M. *Mortally Wounded*. New York, NY: Simon & Schuster, 1996.

37. Martins L. The silence of God: the absence of healing. In: Cox GR, Fundis RJ, eds. *Spiritual, Ethical and Pastoral Aspects of Death and Bereavement*. Amityville, NY: Baywood Publishing; 1992:25–31.

38. Pellegrino E, Thomasma D. *The Christian Virtues in Medical Practice*. Washington, DC: Georgetown University Press; 1996.

39. Germino BB, Fife BL, Funk SG. Cancer and the partner relationship: what is its meaning? *Semin Oncol Nurs.* 1995;11(1):43–50.

40. Bowman T. Facing loss of dreams: A special kind of grief. *Int J Palliat Nurs.* 1997;3(2):76–80.

41. Garbarino J. The spiritual challenge of violent trauma. *Am J Orthopsychiatry.* 1996;66(1):162–163.

42. Rando TA. *Treatment of Complicated Mourning*. Champaign, IL: Research Press; 1993.

43. Kallenberg K. Is there meaning in suffering? An external question in a new context. Paper presented at: Cancer Nursing Changing Frontiers; 1992; Vienna, Austria.

44. American Nurses Association. Provision 1.3: The nature of health problems. In: *American Nurses Association Code of Ethics for Nurses with Interpretive Statements*. Silver Spring, MD: American Nurses Publishing, 2011. http://www.nursingworld.org/provision-1. Accessed April 4, 2015.

45. Kahn DL, Steeves RH. The significance of suffering in cancer care. *Semin Oncol Nurs.* 1995;11(1):9–16.

46. Byock I. When suffering persists. *J Pall Care.* 1994;10(2):8–13.

47. Kuhl D. What dying people want. In: Chochinov H, Breitbart W, eds. *Handbook of Psychiatry in Palliative Medicine*. New York, NY: Oxford University Press; 2009:141–156.

48. Downey L, Engelberg RA, Curtis JR, Lafferty WE, Patrick DL. Shared priorities for the end-of-life period. *J Pain Symptom Manage.* 2009;37(2):175–188.

49. Bailey SS. The arts in spiritual care. *Semin Oncol Nurs.* 1997;13(4):242–247.

50. Baldacchino D, Draper P. Spiritual coping strategies: a review of the nursing research literature. *J Adv Nurs.* 2001;34(6):833–841.

51. Sellers SC. The spiritual care meanings of adults residing in the midwest. *Nurs Sci Q.* 2001;14(3):239–248.

52. Zhang B, Nilsson ME, Prigerson HG. Factors important to patients' quality of life at the end of life. *Arch Intern Med.* 2012;172(15):1133–1142.

53. van Uden-Kraan CF, Chinapaw MJ, Drossaert CH, Verdonck-de Leeuw IM, Buffart LM. Cancer patients' experiences with and perceived outcomes of yoga: results from focus groups. *Support Care Cancer.* 2013;21(7):1861–1870.

54. Albaugh JA. Spirituality and life-threatening illness: a phenomenologic study. *Oncol Nurs Forum.* 2003;30(4):593–598.

55. Taylor EJ. Nurses caring for the spirit: patients with cancer and family caregiver expectations. *Oncol Nurs Forum.* 2003;30(4):585–590.

56. Smith AR, DeSanto-Madeya S, Perez JE, et al.: How women with advanced cancer pray: a report from two focus groups. *Oncol Nurs Forum.* 2012;39(3):E310–E316.

57. Kaut K. Religion, spirituality, and existentialism near the end of life. *Am Behav Scientist.* 2002;46(2):220–234.

58. Ressler PK, Bradshaw YS, Gualtieri L, Chui KK. Communicating the experience of chronic pain and illness through blogging. *J Med Internet Res* 2012;14(5):e143.

59. Keim-Malpass J, Steeves RH. Talking with death at a diner: young women's online narratives of cancer. *Oncol Nurs Forum.* 2012;39(4):373–378, 406.

60. McClement S, Chochinov H. Hope in advanced cancer patients. *Eur J Cancer.* 2008;44(8):1169–1174.

61. Balvere P, Cassessl J, Buzaianu E. Professional nursing burnout and irrational thinking. *J Nurs Staff Dev.* 2012;28(1):2–8.

62. Epstein EG, Hamric AB: Moral distress, moral residue, and the crescendo effect. *J Clin Ethics* 2009;20(4):330–342.

63. Hamric AB: Empirical research on moral distress: issues, challenges, and opportunities. *HEC Forum* 2012;24(1):39–49.

64. Albom M: *Tuesdays With Morrie.* New York, NY: Doubleday; 1997.

Chapter 5

The Meaning of Hope in the Dying

Valerie T. Cotter and Anessa M. Foxwell

Hope is a powerful influence in our lives. Hope is potentially everywhere, including the bedside of someone who is dying. When mobilized effectively, robust hope is precious; when left untended, effete hope can send us in perilous directions.[1]

Hope has long been recognized as fundamental to the human experience. Many authors have contemplated hope, extolling it as a virtue and an energy that brings life and joy.[2-4] Fromm[2] called hope "a psychic commitment to life and growth." Some authors assert that life without hope is impossible.[4]

Despite its positive connotations, hope is intimately bound with loss and suffering. As the French philosopher Gabriel Marcel[3] observed, "Hope is situated within the framework of the trial." It is this paradox that manifests itself so fully at the end of life.

Indeed, the critical role that hope plays in human life takes on special meaning as death nears. The ability to hope often is challenged, and it can elude patients and families during terminal illness. Hope for a cure is almost certainly destroyed, and even a prolonged reprieve from death is unlikely. Many patients and families experience multiple losses as they continue an illness trajectory marked by increasing disability and pain.

Even when hope appears to be strong within the dying person or the family, it can be problematic if hopefulness is perceived to be based on unrealistic ideas about the future.[5,6] Tension grows within relationships as people become absorbed in a struggle between competing versions of reality. Important issues may be left unresolved as individuals continue to deny the reality of impending death.

Despite these somber realities and the inevitable suffering, many people do maintain hope as they die, and families recover and find hope even within the experience of loss. How can this be? Part of the reason lies in the nature of hope itself—its resiliency and capacity to coexist with suffering. As witnesses to suffering and hope, palliative care nurses must understand these complexities and be confident and sensitive in their efforts to address hope and hopelessness in the people for whom they care.

To assist palliative care nurses, this chapter explores the many dimensions of hope and identifies its possible influence on health and quality of life. Nursing assessment and strategies to foster hope are described. In addition, specific issues such as "unrealistic hopefulness" and cultural considerations in the expression and maintenance of hope are discussed. The goals of the chapter are to provide the reader with an understanding of this complex but vital phenomenon; to offer guidance in the clinical application of this concept to palliative nursing care; and to explore some of the controversies about hope that challenge clinicians.

Definitions and Dimensions of Hope

Hope is an important concept for many disciplines, including philosophy, theology, psychology, nursing, and medicine. A classic nursing theory of hope, developed by Karin Dufault,[7] is particularly notable in its comprehensiveness. Dufault[7] described hope as "a multidimensional, dynamic life force characterized by a confident yet uncertain expectation of achieving a future good which, to the hoping person, is realistically possible and personally significant." Dufault also theorized that hope has two interrelated spheres: particularized and generalized. *Particularized hope* is centered and dependent on specific valued goals or hope objects. An example is the hope of a terminally ill patient to live long enough to celebrate a particular holiday or event. In contrast, *generalized hope* is a broader, nonspecific sense of a more positive future that is not directly related to a particular goal or desire. Dufault likened this sphere to an umbrella that creates a diffuse, positive glow on life.

Dufault postulated six dimensions of hope: affective, spiritual, relational, cognitive, behavioral, and contextual. The *affective* dimension of hope encompasses a myriad of emotions. Of course, hope is accompanied by many positive feelings, including joy, confidence, strength, and excitement. The full experience of hope, however, also includes uncertainty, fear, anger, suffering, and sometimes despair.[8-11] For example, Marcel argued that in its fullest sense hope could only follow an experience of suffering or trial.[3] Marcel's thesis is corroborated by the experiences described by people with cancer who see their disease as "a wake-up call" that has opened their eyes to a greater appreciation for life and an opportunity for self-growth—in other words, an event that has forced them to confront their mortality while also inspiring hope.[15] The *spiritual* dimension is a central component of hope.[12-15] Hopefulness is associated with spiritual well-being,[13,16,17] and qualitative studies have shown that spirituality and spiritual practices provide a context in which to define hope and articulate hope-fostering activities.[7,18] These activities include religious beliefs and rituals but extend to broader conceptualizations of spirituality that encompass meaning and purpose in life, self-transcendence, and connectedness with a deity or other life force.[14,19] Although spirituality is almost always viewed as a hope-fostering influence, serious illness and suffering can challenge one's belief and trust in a benevolent deity, or be viewed as punishment from God; either interpretation of suffering can result in hopelessness. [20]

Relationships with significant others are another important dimension of hope. Interconnectedness with others is cited as a source of hope in virtually every study, and physical and psychological isolation from others is a frequent threat to hope.[12,21,22] Hope levels are positively associated with social support.[23,24] In addition to family members and friends, nurses offer patients a unique and independent source of support for hope. [25,26] Harris et al.[21] reported that HIV peer-counseling relationships inspired hope in both the counseling recipients and their counselors. Despite being vital sources of hope, other people can threaten a patient's hope by distancing themselves from the patient, showing disrespect, discounting the patient's experiences, disclosing negative information, or withholding information.[20,22]

The *cognitive* dimension of hope encompasses many intellectual strategies, particularly those involving specific goals that require planning and effort to attain. Identifying goals can motivate and energize people, thereby increasing hope.[21,27] When identifying goals, people assess what they desire and value within a context of what is realistically possible.[28] They appraise the resources necessary to accomplish their goals against the resources that are available to them. They then take action to secure the resources or meet the goals, and they decide on a reasonable time frame in which to accomplish the goals.[29] Active involvement in one's situation and attainment of goals increases the sense of personal control and self-efficacy, which, in turn, increases hope.[28] If a person repeatedly fails to attain valued goals, hopelessness and negative emotions, such as anxiety, depression, or anger, can result.[27]

The *behavioral,* goal-focused thoughts and activities that foster hope are similar to the problem-focused coping strategies originally described by Lazarus and Folkman.[30] This similarity is not surprising, because hope is strongly associated with coping.[31] Hope has been identified as a foundation or mediator for successful coping, a method of coping, and an outcome of successful coping.[31,32] Many strategies that people use to maintain hope have been identified previously as coping methods, and models of maintaining hope overlap substantially with models of coping.[5,31] Strategies to maintain hope include problem-focused coping methods (e.g., setting goals, actively managing symptoms, getting one's affairs in order) and emotion-focused strategies (e.g., using distraction techniques, appraising the illness in non-threatening ways).[5,31,33]

Contextual dimensions of hope are the life circumstances and abilities that influence hope—for example, physical health, financial stability, and functional and cognitive abilities. Common threats to hope include acute, chronic, and terminal illness; cognitive decline; fatigue; pain; and impaired functional status.[31,34] These factors, particularly physical illness and impairment, do not inevitably decrease hope if people are able to overcome the threat through cognitive, spiritual, relational, or other strategies.

Influence of Hope and Hopelessness on Adaptation to Illness

Hope influences health and adaptation to illness. Empirical evidence indicates that diminished hope is associated with poorer quality of life,[32] persistence of suicidal ideation,[35] and higher incidence of suicide.[36] Hopelessness also increases the likelihood that people will consider physician-assisted death as an option for themselves[37] Hopelessness is significant in the etiology and maintenance of depression. [36]

In addition to its influence on psychological states and behaviors, there is some evidence to suggest that hope affects physical states as well. Researchers have found associations between hopelessness and early markers of endothelial dysfunction, a precursor to atherosclerosis.[38] Rawdin and colleagues[34] reported that hope was associated with the psychosocial elements of the pain experience.

Variations in Hope Among Different Populations

The preceding description of hope is derived from studies involving diverse populations, including children and older adults. In addition, research has been conducted in inpatient, outpatient, and community settings with well persons and those with a variety of chronic and life-threatening illnesses. The experiences of families also have been described. Over these diverse populations and settings, many core concepts have been identified that transcend specific groups. However, some subtle but important differences exist. For this reason, hopefulness in selected populations is addressed in the following sections.

Hope in Children and their Parents

A few investigators have examined hope in children and their parents. Kylma and Juvakka[39] studied hope in parents of adolescents with cancer. The findings suggested that hope appears to be central to parents who have a child with cancer. Their hope reflected an orientation toward life and the future, trust, connection with others, and wishes. Factors endangering parental hope were related to the adolescent's cancer and deteriorating health status, negative aspects in care received, poor parental resources, tightened economic situation, and other people's negative reactions. Hope-engendering factors were related to the adolescent's constructive personality, positive consequences from adolescent's cancer, adolescent's improving health status, good care, gradual ability to continue life, good parental resources, other people's positive reactions, having faith, and having family pets.

Salmon and colleagues[40] explored how hope arose in interactions between oncologists and parents of children aged 1 to 12 years with acute lymphoblastic leukemia. The investigators found an interpersonal basis of hope (e.g., most parents linked their ability to hope to "having faith in" the oncologist and consistently valued oncologists' explicit positivity) and a psychological basis of hope (e.g., focusing on short-term events associated with treatment and avoiding information about the longer term).

In another study, Mack and colleagues[41] surveyed parents of children with cancer and the children's physicians to evaluate relationships between parental recall of prognostic disclosure by the physician and possible outcomes, including hope, trust, and emotional distress. Nearly half of parents reported that physician communication always made them feel hopeful. Parents were more likely to report communication-related hope when they also recalled increased prognostic disclosure.

Hope and Older Adults

Numerous studies have examined hope in ill and healthy older adults.[42-44] Findings from these studies suggest that certain hope-related themes and factors take on special significance for this age group. For example, in a recent metasynthesis of qualitative research, hope was described as an important psychological resource that helped older adults deal with chronic illness.[43] Older adults used two interrelated processes to help deal with their experience: (1) transcendence, a process of reaching inwardly and outwardly, and finding meaning and purpose; and (2) positive reappraisal, a recognition and acknowledgment that their situation had changed and they could see positive possibilities for the future. Although chronic illness that impairs physical functioning is linked with decreased hope, diagnosis of a life-threatening disease such as cancer is not associated with low levels of hope.[45] This finding may reflect an attitude among older adults that the quality of life that remains matters more than the quantity.

Hirsch and colleagues[42] studied older adults recruited from primary care settings. They found that functional impairment was associated with increased depressive symptoms, and individuals with higher levels of hope experienced fewer depressive symptoms. Also, the ability to generate goals and resources to accomplish goals contributed to higher levels of hope.

Among younger European American adults, hope tends to be tied to being productive; personal and professional achievements figure prominently in one's ability to nurture and maintain hope. In contrast, older adults are more likely to focus on spirituality, relationships, leaving a legacy focused on others, and other factors that are not linked with accomplishment.[46] Hope-fostering activities include reminiscing, controlling symptoms, spirituality, and connecting with others.

Hope From the Family Caregiver's Perspective

Family caregivers are an integral component in palliative care. Patients and families influence each other's hope, and nursing interventions must focus on both groups. Often, the physical and psychological demands placed on family caregivers are great, as are threats to hope.[33,47,48] Threats to hope in caregivers include isolation from support networks, questioning of one's spiritual beliefs; concurrent losses, including loss of significant others, health, and income; and inability to control the patient's symptoms. Holtslander and Duggleby[49] reported that difficulties in communicating with healthcare providers, feelings of depersonalization, and receipt of "too many negative messages" also eroded caregivers' hope. Other studies found that hope played a significant role in family caregivers' perception of increased strain and overall quality of life.[50,51]

Strategies to maintain hope in family caregivers are similar to those found in patients, with a few differences. Spending time with others in the support network was very important for caregivers. In addition, being able to reprioritize demands helped caregivers conserve much-needed energy. Obtaining respite from the caregiving role also promoted hope.[49]

Caregiver Hope in Metastatic Cancer—A Story

Mr. R, a 64-year-old married man and retired auditor, was recently diagnosed with metastatic non–small-cell lung cancer. Nine months prior, Mr. R began experiencing right shoulder pain while playing golf. He sought treatment from multiple providers including an internist, an orthopedist, three different pain specialists, a physical therapist, a chiropractor, and an acupuncturist. Most of these practitioners believed Mr. R to be suffering from a torn rotator cuff, until he was evaluated for right hand weakness by a neurologist who ordered an MRI and found a right apical lung mass. When Mr. R retired from a demanding job last year, he and his wife moved into a retirement community complete with amenities including a golf course. Mr. R promised his wife he would spend more time with their grandchildren and quit smoking, as his daily stress diminished. The couple enjoyed their time together until Mr. R's undiagnosed pain and many appointments added frustration and heartache.

After finally meeting with an oncologist and receiving a definitive diagnosis, Mr. R began palliative radiation to right clavicle metastases. A week later Mr. R's mobility and pain improved. As his primary caregiver, Mrs. R's hope developed, as she had answers and a treatment plan. Mrs. R contacted the American Cancer Society and inquired about nearby caregiver support groups. The couple completed their advance directives together and began working to update financial and other paperwork. Mrs. R admitted feeling overwhelmed at times by the process to get their affairs in order while keeping up with housework. Mrs. R was grateful to be living in a very supportive retirement community, where one neighbor cooked a weekly meal for them and another knitted Mr. R a prayer shawl. Mr. & Mrs. R's hope was influenced by the possibility of a cure and the drive to remain strong for their children and grandchildren. Mrs. R found comfort and solace in the community pool, swimming as a cathartic outlet.

Hope in Terminally Ill Patients: Is Hope Compatible With Death?

Research demonstrates that many people are able to maintain hope during acute and chronic illness. Hope also can thrive during the terminal phase of

> **Box 5.1 Sources of Hope/Hope-Fostering Strategies in Terminally Ill Adults**
>
> - Love of family and friends
> - Spirituality/having faith
> - Setting goals and maintaining independence
> - Positive relationships with professional carers
> - Humor
> - Personal characteristics
> - Uplifting memories
>
> Adapted from Buckley J, Herth K. Fostering hope in terminally ill patients. *Nurs Standard*. 2004;19(10):33–41.

an illness, despite the realization that no cure is possible. In qualitative studies, hope was essential to human existence, as integral to life, even when dying.[52,53]

Although hope levels may not decrease, the nature of hope often is altered through the dying process. Other changes in hope at the end of life include an increased focus on relationships and trusting in others, as well as a desire to leave a legacy and to be well remembered.[7,33,46] Spirituality also increases in importance for some patients during the terminal phases of illness.[33] People also adopt specific strategies to foster hope at the end of life.[53,54] Many of these approaches are summarized in Box 5.1.

Although hope tends to change in people with terminal illness, maintaining a delicate balance between acceptance of death and hope for a cure often remains an important task up until the time of death, even when people acknowledge that cure is virtually impossible.[33,54] The dying person needs to envision future moments of happiness, fulfillment, and connection.[52,53]

A Story of Hope Transformed

Mr. S, a 62-year-old Jamaican gentleman, was diagnosed with gastric cancer 5 months ago and has now been admitted to the hospital with increasing abdominal distension and worsening pain at the J-tube site. Just a week prior to his admission, Mr. S had an appointment with his oncologist, who told him that imaging revealed progression of his disease and palliative chemotherapy was recommended. Mr. S refused chemotherapy, as he was worried that his body could not handle further treatment, and he would instead pursue herbal remedies. Mr. S also told his oncologist that perhaps the scans are evidence that his cancer is "breaking up" and he was hopeful that with prayer, a miracle would happen.

Upon admission to the hospital, the primary team felt that Mr. S was in denial and/or did not understand the gravity of his circumstances. Thus, the primary team consulted the Palliative Care Service to help determine goals of care. Mr. S was followed by the interdisciplinary palliative care team, including a spiritual care provider, who was essential in uncovering his hopes for the future. Three years ago, Mr. S battled colon cancer and has been in remission since a surgical resection. Spirituality has guided Mr. S throughout his life, and God, as "the ultimate physician and healer," continued to provide Mr. S with hope. Mr. S prayed and hoped that his cancer was breaking up because he did not feel as though his work was done. Mr. S looked to his four daughters for support and lived with two of them.

Mr. S hoped that he would return to Jamaica to see the birth of his first grandchild in the upcoming month. Mr. S continued to work toward achieving these goals while his symptoms worsened and he eventually transitioned to inpatient hospice care. During his last weeks, Mr. S spent time with his family, shared prayers with trusted chaplains, and filmed a legacy video for his unborn grandson. Although an ultimate hope for a miracle remained, Mr. S acquired new hopes at the end of his life through reflection that led to great comfort and peace for his family.

Multicultural Views of Hope

Over the past three decades, understanding of the clinical phenomenon of hope has increased dramatically through theoretical discourse and empirical investigation. Although knowledge regarding the components, processes, and outcomes of hope has grown, progress in multicultural research on hope has been limited. The samples in many studies that examine hope or hopelessness are ethnically homogeneous,[34,46,55] or their ethnic composition is unknown.[32,50] The studies that do include ethnically diverse samples are small,[56,57] precluding any comparisons or generalization of findings.

Several excellent European studies have contributed greatly to the general understanding of hope.[9,10,29,40] However, many of these investigations use frameworks and instruments developed by US researchers whose work is founded on homogeneous samples. Moreover, it may be that hopefulness for Europeans is more similar to that of middle-class Americans than it is different from them.[33]

Farone and colleagues[58] examined the associations among locus of control, negative affect, hope, and self-reported health in 109 older Mexican American women with cancer. They found that hope and internal locus of control both showed significant associations with better health outcomes. Although these findings are similar to those for white non-Hispanic samples, the authors cautioned that they were unable to explore the characteristics of control that may be unique to Latina populations. They recommended that future research include attribution of control based on religious beliefs and the concept of *fatalismo* (fatalism).

Despite the growing body of research in diverse samples, existing research may not adequately reflect the experience of hope for people from non-European cultures. Several known cultural differences could certainly limit the applicability of current conceptualizations of hope, especially within the palliative care context. Three issues that theoretically could have a major impact on multicultural views of hope are time orientation, truth-telling, and one's beliefs about control.

Time orientation is identified as a cultural phenomenon that varies among cultural groups. Some cultural groups, usually highly individualistic ones, are future-oriented. Within these groups, people prefer to look ahead, make short- and long-term plans, and organize their schedules to meet goals.[59] Because hope is defined as being future-oriented, with hopeful people more likely to identify and take action to meet goals, members of these future-oriented cultures may possibly appear more hopeful than people who are predominantly present-focused. On the other hand, people who are more focused on the present may be better able to sustain hope at the end of life, when the ability to create long-range goals is hindered by the uncertainty surrounding a terminal diagnosis. Additional research is needed to clarify these relationships.

The value for truth-telling in Western healthcare systems also may affect hope. Current ethical and legal standards require full disclosure of all relevant healthcare information to patients.[60] Informed consent and patient autonomy in medical decision-making, two eminent values in American healthcare, are impossible without this disclosure.[60] Although few would advocate lying to patients, truth-telling is not universally viewed as helpful or desirable.[61,62] In some cultures, it is believed that patients should be protected from burdensome information that could threaten hope. Truthful but blunt communication may also be seen as rude and disrespectful in some cultures, and the feeling of being devalued and disrespected has a negative impact on hope. In addition to the threats to hope that frank discussion is believed to engender, people who prefer nondisclosure of threatening information may be seen as attempting to cling to unrealistic hopes by refusing to listen to discouraging facts about their condition.

A third cultural concept that may affect hope is one's feeling of being in control. Control is a core attribute in many conceptualizations of hope. Although control can be relinquished to others, including healthcare providers or a transcendent power, personal control often is central to the hoping process. In Euro-American cultures, applying one's will and energy to alter the course of an illness or to direct the dying process seems natural and desirable. Advance directives are one culturally sanctioned way in which members of these societies exert control over the dying process.[63] However, this desire for and belief in personal control is not a common feature in many other cultures. In cultures where death is viewed as part of the inherent harmony of living and dying, attempts to exert any influence over the dying process may seem unnatural or inappropriate.[63] People from diverse cultures who take a more passive role in their healthcare, or who do not espouse a desire to control their illness or the dying process, may be viewed as less hopeful than people who manifest a "fighting spirit" and active stance.

More research is needed to test theories of hope in multicultural groups, both to ensure the appropriate application of current conceptualizations to diverse cultural groups, and to develop new theories that are relevant for these groups. Until this work is done, palliative care clinicians must be cautious in applying current hope theories, and be sensitive to the possible variations in diverse populations.

Models of Maintaining Hope for People With Life-Threatening Illnesses

Many investigators have identified factors that foster hope, and strategies that enable people to sustain hope despite life-threatening or chronic illness. Although there is considerable concordance across these studies regarding many of the major themes, various models emphasize different styles and strategies that demonstrate the diversity in hope-fostering approaches.

Many people with terminal illness turn to activities and coping strategies that cultivate generalized hope rather than an emphasis on achievement and control. These strategies reflect a sense of peace and acceptance of death, and center on "being" rather than "doing." These strategies are described in Box 5.1.

In contrast, Olsson and colleagues found that patients preserved their hope using two goal-oriented or problem solving processes: (1) maintaining life and (2) preparing for death. The patients tried to maintain life in several ways by keeping up with their day-to-day tasks and hobbies; communicating with others about practical matters and emotional feelings; involving other people such as family, friends or professionals; and actively searching elsewhere for something to give them hope. To prepare for death, patients took responsibility for planning their own funeral and other practical matters, and arranged things so their family would have less of a burden. People use multiple strategies that allow them to confront and avoid the negative aspects of illness and death. Although the strategies used to manage the threat of death often seem to predominate, these activities occur within a background of recognition and acknowledgment of the possibility of death. This process of negotiating between acknowledgment and management of these fears has been identified in other studies of people with life-threatening illnesses.[8]

Although some people continue to search for a cure after receiving a terminal diagnosis, hoping for a cure can coexist with awareness of death and engagement with life's activities.[53] Most people eventually accept their prognosis and mourn the loss of their original goals. At this point, they need to develop and pursue alternative goals that are possible in light of their diminished physical function, end of life symptoms, and loss of energy.

These different approaches for maintaining hope are important to describe and understand because they assist the palliative care nurse in designing effective strategies to foster hope. They increase clinicians' awareness regarding the various ways that people respond to chronic and terminal illness, and guide clinicians in their interactions with patients and families to sustain hope. They also help palliative care providers understand difficult or troubling responses, such as unrealistic hopefulness.

The Issue of "Unrealistic" Hopefulness

Reality surveillance is a feature of many conceptualizations of hope. Often, clinicians, researchers, and theorists believe that mentally healthy people should choose and work toward realistic goals. In these frameworks, adhering to unrealistic hopes or denying reality is a sign of maladaptive cognitions that could lead to negative health outcomes. Therefore, denial and unrealistic hopes and ideas are discouraged and treated as pathological.[5,6]

Clinical examples of unrealistic hopes that cause consternation are numerous and diverse. For instance, one patient with advanced cancer might hope that his persistent severe sciatica is from exercise and overuse rather than spinal metastases. The nurse working with this patient may continually contradict his theory, asserting that his denial of the probable malignant cause of the pain will delay effective treatment. Another patient might insist that a new cure for her illness is imminent, causing distress for the nurse, who believes that the patient's unrealistic hopes will hinder acceptance of and preparation for death.

Despite these concerns, however, some investigators argue that the nurses' fears may be unfounded. This perspective is based on more recent studies, which have led researchers to question the view that denial and unrealistic hopes are maladaptive. Instead, they argue that to maintain that these patients are professing unrealistic hopes is to challenge or negate the legitimacy of the dominant depiction of the promise and potential cure provided by medical science.[52,53] Eliott and Olver[52] suggest that clinicians should not be concerned whether hope is real or unreal, true or false, present or not; rather they should view hope as an attempt to articulate, share, and value with others those things that connect the patient to what give their lives meaning, and ultimately, to life (pp. 148).

In addition to promoting positive outcomes, "unrealistic" hopes need to be assessed within the context of uncertainty. For instance, people frequently respond to dire prognostic news with the observation that they can always "beat the odds." Given that no one can predict the future with absolute certainty, it is impossible to predict which individuals with a 2% chance of remission or recovery will actually be cured. So, if a person hopes for something in the future that appears highly unlikely, can it be known for certain that it will not occur? Patients and families often need to focus on this uncertainty to sustain hope.[8] Research supports the idea that patients' and families' hopes and goals are effective coping strategies, even when the likelihood of obtaining them seems remote. [51,53]

Olsman and colleagues[64] conducted an interpretative synthesis of the literature showing that nurses and physicians could take three perspectives with hope of palliative care patients: (1) realistic perspective, (2) functional perspective, and (3) narrative perspective. Clinicians view hope from a realistic perspective when that hope is truthful and when the "truth" is adjusted to the reality. From a functional perspective, hope helps patients cope with treatments or face uncertainty. Nurses who take a narrative perspective focus on the meaning that is valuable to patients. Olsman and colleagues also suggested that clinicians can take more than one perspective at the same time.

Assessing Hope

As in all nursing care, thorough assessment of physical and psychosocial factors must precede thoughtful planning and implementation of therapeutic strategies. Therefore, consistent and comprehensive evaluations of hope should be included in the palliative nursing assessment. Some conceptual elements of hope, such as those focusing on meaning and purpose in life, are included in a spiritual assessment. Rarely, however, are comprehensive guides to assessing hope included in standardized nursing assessment forms.

The guidelines produced by Farran, Wilken, and Popovich[65] for the clinical assessment of hope appropriately use the acronym HOPE to designate the major areas of evaluation: Health, Others, Purpose in Life, and Engaging Process. The term *Engaging Process* refers to identifying goals, taking actions to achieve goals, sense of control over one's situation, and identifying hope-inspiring factors in one's past, present, and future. In Table 5.1, this

Table 5.1 Guidelines for the Clinical Assessment of Hope in Palliative Care	
Interview Question/Probe	**Rationale**
Health (and symptom management)	
1. Tell me about your illness. What is your understanding of the probable course of your illness?	Explore the person's perceptions of seriousness of his or her illness, and possible trajectories
2. How hopeful are you right now, and how does your illness affect your sense of hope?	Determine the person's general sense of hope and the effect of the terminal illness on hope
3. How well are you able to control the symptoms of your illness? How do these symptoms affect your hope?	Uncontrolled end of life symptoms have been found to negatively influence hope
Others	
1. Who provides you with emotional, physical, and spiritual support?	Identify people in the environment that provide support and enhance hope
2. Who are you most likely to confide in when you have a problem or concern?	Identify others in whom the person has trust
3. What kinds of difficult experiences have you and your family/partner/ support network had to deal with in the past? How did you manage those experiences?	Explore experiences of coping with stressful situations
4. What kinds of things do family, support people, and healthcare providers do that make you more hopeful? Less hopeful?	Identify specific behaviors that affect hope and recognize that other people can also decrease hope
Purpose in life	
1. What gives you hope?	Identify relationships, beliefs, and activities that provide a sense of purpose and contribute positively to hope

(continued)

Table 5.1 (Continued)

Interview Question/Probe	Rationale
2. What helps you make sense of your situation right now?	Identify the ways in which the person makes meaning of difficult situations.
3. Do you have spiritual or religious practices or support people who help you? If "yes," what are these practices or people?	Identify if and how spirituality acts as a source of hope
4. Has your illness caused you to question your spiritual beliefs? If "yes," how?	Terminal illness can threaten the person's basic beliefs and test one's faith
5. How can we help you maintain these practices and personal connections with spiritual support people?	Identify ways in which clinicians and others can support spiritual practices that enhance hope
Goals	
1. Right now, what are your major goals?	Identify major goals and priorities
	Examine whether these goals are congruent with the views of others
2. What do you see are the chances that you will meet these goals?	Explore how realistic the person thinks the goals are; if the goals are not perceived as being attainable, assess the impact on hope
3. What actions can you take to meet these goals?	Identify specific actions the person can take to meet the goals
4. What actions have you already taken to meet these goals?	Identify how active the person has been in attaining the goals
5. What resources do you have for meeting these goals?	Determine other resources to which the person has access for the purpose of attaining goals
Sense of control	
1. Do you feel that you have much control over your current situation?	Determine if the person feels any ability to control or change the situation
	Explore whether the person wants to have more control
2. Are there others that you feel have some control over your current situation? If "yes," who are they and in what ways do they have control?	Determine if the person feels as though trusted others (e.g., healthcare providers, family, deity) can control or change the situation
Sources of hope over time	
1. In the past, what or who has made you hopeful?	Identify sources of hope from the person's past that may continue to provide hope during the terminal phase
2. Right now who and what provides you with hope?	Identify current sources of hope
3. What do you hope for in the future?	Assess generalized and specific hopes for the future

Adapted from Farran CJ, Wilken C, Popovich JM. Clinical assessment of hope. *Issues Ment Health Nurs.* 1992;13(2):129–138 and Farran CJ, Herth KA, Popovich JM. *Hope and Hopelessness: Critical Clinical Constructs.* Thousand Oaks, CA: SAGE; 1995.

framework has been adapted and applied to terminally ill patients. It includes examples of questions and probes that can be used to assess hope.

Like pain, hope is a subjective experience and assessment should focus on self-report. However, behavioral cues can also provide information regarding a person's state of hope or hopelessness. Hopelessness is a central feature of depression; therefore, behaviors such as social withdrawal, flat affect, alcohol and substance abuse, insomnia, and passivity may indicate hopelessness.

As discussed in the "Hope From the Family Caregiver's Perspective" section, the patient's terminal illness affects the hope of family caregivers, who, in turn, influence the hope of the patients. Therefore, the hope of the patient's family caregivers and other significant support people also should be assessed.

Over the past decades, researchers from several disciplines have developed instruments to measure hope and hopelessness. The theoretical and empirical literature documents the comprehensiveness and face validity of these tools. Advances in psychometric theory and methods have allowed the evaluation of multiple dimensions of validity and reliability. The development and use of well-designed and well-tested tools has contributed greatly to the science of hope. Although a thorough discussion of these measures is beyond the scope of this chapter, Table 5.2 provides a brief description of several widely used and tested instruments.

Nursing Interventions to Maintain Hope at End of Life

Clinicians, theorists, and researchers recognize that nurses play an important role in instilling, maintaining, and restoring hope in people for whom they care. Researchers have identified many ways in which nurses assist patients and families to sustain hope in the face of life-threatening illness. Box 5.2 provides a summary of nursing approaches to instill hope. A brief perusal of this table reveals an important point about these strategies: For the most part, nursing care to maintain patients' and families' hope is fundamentally about providing excellent physical, psychosocial, and spiritual palliative care. There are few unique interventions to maintain hope, and yet there is much nurses can do. Because hope is inextricably connected to virtually all facets of the illness experience—including physical pain, coping, anxiety, and spirituality—improvement or deterioration in one area has repercussions in other areas. Attending to these relationships reminds clinicians that virtually every action they take can influence hope, negatively or positively.

Another vital observation about hope-inspiring strategies is that many approaches begin with the patient and family. The experience of hope is a personal one, defined and determined by the hoping person. Although others greatly influence that experience, ultimately the meanings and effects of words and actions are determined by the person experiencing hope or hopelessness. Many approaches used by people with life-threatening illness to maintain hope are strategies initiated with little influence from others. For example, some people pray; others distract themselves with television watching, conversation, or other activities; and many patients use cognitive strategies, such as minimizing negative thoughts, identifying personal strengths, and focusing on the positive. For many patients and families, careful observation

Table 5.2 Descriptions of Selected Instruments to Measure Hope and Hopelessness

Instrument Name	Brief Description
Beck Hopelessness Scale	• 20-item, true-false format
	• Based on Stotland's definition of hopelessness: system of negative expectancies concerning oneself and one's future
	• Developed to assess psychopathological levels of hopelessness; correlates highly with attempted and actual suicide
Herth Hope Index	• 12-item, 4-point Likert scale; total score is sum of all items; range of scores 12–48
	• Designed for well and ill populations
	• Assesses three overlapping dimensions: (1) cognitive-temporal, (2) affective-behavioral, (3) affiliative-behavioral
	• Spanish, Thai, Chinese, Swedish translations available
Hopefulness Scale for Adolescents (Hinds)	• 24-item visual analog scale
	• Assesses the degree of the adolescent's positive future orientation
	• Assesses only the relational and rational thoughts processes of hope
	• Tested in several populations of adolescents: well, substance abusers, adolescents with emotional and mental problems, cancer patients
Miller Hope Scale	• 40-item scale, 5-point Likert scale
	• Assesses 10 elements: (a) mutuality/affiliation, (b) avoidance of absolutizing, (c) sense of the possible, (d) psychological well-being and coping, (e) achieving goals, (f) purpose and meaning in life, (g) reality surveillance-optimism, (h) mental and physical activation, (i) anticipation, (j) freedom
	• Chinese and Swedish versions
Snyder Hope Scale	• 12-item, 4-point Likert scale
	• Based on Stotland's definition of hope; focus is on goals identification and achievement
	• Tested in healthy adults, and adults with psychiatric illness
	• Also has developed tool to measure hope in children

and active support of an individual's established strategies to maintain hope will be most successful.

Family caregivers and other support people should be included in these approaches. Ample evidence demonstrates that patients and people within their support systems reciprocally influence one another's hope. In addition,

Box 5.2 Nursing Actions to Foster Hope

Experiential Processes

- Prevent and manage end of life symptoms
- Use lightheartedness and humor appropriately
- Encourage the patient and family to transcend their current situation
- Encourage aesthetic experiences
- Encourage engagement in creative and joyous endeavors
- Suggest literature, movies, and art that are uplifting and highlight the joy in life
- Encourage reminiscing
- Assist patient and family to focus on present and past joys
- Share positive, hope-inspiring stories
- Support patient and family in positive self-talk

Spiritual/Transcendent Processes

- Facilitate participation in religious rituals and spiritual practices
- Make necessary referrals to clergy and other spiritual support people
- Assist the patient and family in finding meaning in the current situation
- Assist the patient/family in keeping a journal
- Suggest literature, movies, and art that explore the meaning of suffering

Relational Processes

- Minimize patient and family isolation
- Establish and maintain an open relationship
- Affirm patients' and families' sense of self-worth
- Recognize and reinforce the reciprocal nature of hopefulness between patient and support system
- Provide time for relationships (especially important in institutional settings)
- Foster attachment ideation by assisting the patient to identify significant others and then to reflect on personal characteristics and experiences that endear the significant other to the patient
- Communicate one's own sense of hopefulness

Rational Thought Processes

- Assist patient and family to establish, obtain, and revise goals without imposing one's own agenda
- Assist in identifying available and needed resources to meet goals
- Assist in procuring needed resources; assist with breaking larger goals into smaller steps to increase feelings of success
- Provide accurate information regarding patient's condition and treatment in a skillful and sensitive manner
- Help patient and family identify past successes
- Increase patients' and families' sense of control when possible

family and significant others are always incorporated into the palliative care plan and considered part of the unit of care. Maintenance of hope also is a goal after death, in that hope-restoring and -maintaining strategies must be an integral part of bereavement counseling.[66,67]

Specific Interventions

The framework for the following discussion is adapted from Farran, Herth, and Popovich,[68] who articulated four central attributes of hope: experiential, spiritual/transcendent, relational, and rational thought. These areas encompass the major themes found in the literature, and although they are not mutually exclusive, they provide a useful organizing device. This section also includes a brief discussion of ways in which nurses need to explore and understand their own hopes and values in order to provide palliative care that fosters hope in others.

Experiential Process Interventions

The experiential process of hope involves the acknowledgment and acceptance of suffering, while using the imagination to move beyond the suffering and find hope.[15] Included in these types of strategies are methods to decrease physical suffering and cognitive strategies aimed at managing the threat of the terminal illness.

Uncontrolled symptoms, such as pain, fatigue, dyspnea, and anxiety, cause suffering and challenge the hopefulness of patients and caregivers. Timely and adept symptom prevention and management is central to maintaining hope. In home-care settings, teaching patients and families the knowledge and skills to manage symptoms confidently and competently also is essential.

Other ways to help people find hope in suffering is to provide them a cognitive reprieve from their situation. One powerful strategy to achieve this temporary suspension is through humor. Humor helps put things in perspective and frees the self, at least momentarily, from the onerous burden of illness and suffering. Making light of a grim situation brings a sense of control over one's response to the situation, even when one has little influence over it. Of course, the use of humor with patients and families requires sensitivity as well as a sense of timing. The nurse should take cues from the patient and family, observe how they use humor to dispel stress, and let them take the lead in joking about threatening information and events. In general, humor should be focused on oneself or on events outside the immediate concerns of the patient and family.

Other ways to move people cognitively beyond their suffering is to assist them in identifying and enjoying that which is joyful in life. Engagement in aesthetic experiences, such as watching movies or listening to uplifting music, can enable people to transcend their suffering. Sharing one's own hope-inspiring stories also can help.

Another strategy is to support people in their own positive self-talk. Often people naturally cope with stress by comparing themselves with people they perceive to be less fortunate or by identifying attributes of personal strength that help them find hope.[21,54] For example, an elderly married woman with advanced breast cancer may comment that, despite the seriousness of her disease, she feels luckier than another woman with the same disease who is younger or without social support. By comparing herself with less fortunate others, she can take solace in recognizing that "things could be worse." Similarly, a person can maintain hope by focusing on particular talents or previous accomplishments that indicate an ability to cope with illness. People may also cite their high level of motivation as a reason to feel hopeful about the future. Acknowledgment and validation of these attributes supports hope and affirms self-worth for patients and families.

Spiritual Process Interventions

Several specific strategies can foster hope while incorporating spirituality. These strategies include providing opportunities for the expression of spiritual beliefs and arranging for involvement in religious rituals and spiritual practices.

Assisting patients and families to explore and make meaning of their trials and suffering is another useful approach. Encouraging patients and families to keep a journal of thoughts and feelings can help people in this process. Suggesting books, films, or art that focuses on religious or existential understanding and transcendence of suffering is another effective way to help people make sense of illness and death.

Palliative care nurses also should assess for signs of spiritual distress and make appropriate referrals to spiritual care providers and other professionals with expertise in counseling during spiritual and existential crises.

Relational Process Interventions

To maximize hope, nurses should establish and maintain an open relationship with patients and members of their support network, taking the time to learn what their priorities and needs are and then addressing those needs in timely, effective ways. Demonstrating respect and interest, and being available to listen and be with people—that is, affirming each person's worth—are essential.

Fostering and sustaining connectedness among the patient, family, and friends can be accomplished by providing time for uninterrupted interactions, which is especially important in institutional settings. Nurses can increase hope by enlisting help from others to achieve goals. For example, recruiting friends or arranging for a volunteer to transport an ill person to purchase a gift for a grandchild can cultivate hope for everyone involved. It is important to help others realize how vital they are in sustaining a person's hope.

Rational Thought Process Interventions

The rational thought process is the dimension of hope that specifically focuses on goals, resources, personal control and self-efficacy, and action. Interventions related to this dimension include assisting patients and families in devising and attaining goals. Providing accurate and timely information about the patient's condition and treatment helps patients and families decide which goals are achievable. At times, gentle assistance with monitoring and acknowledging negative possibilities helps the patient and family to choose realistic goals. Helping to identify and procure the resources necessary to meet goals also is important.

Often, major goals need to be broken into smaller, shorter-term achievements. For example, a patient with painful, metastatic lung cancer might want to attend a family event that is two weeks away. The successful achievement of this goal depends on many factors, including adequate pain control, transportation, and ability to transfer to and from a wheelchair. By breaking the larger goal into several smaller ones, the person is able to identify all the necessary steps and resources. Supporting patients and families to identify those areas of life and death in which they do have real influence can increase self-esteem and self-efficacy, thereby instilling hope. It also helps to review their previous successes in attaining important goals.

This domain also includes ways in which clinicians balance the need to communicate "bad news" while sustaining patients' and families' hope. The difficulties inherent in delivering negative information to patients and families does not release us from our duty to communicate openly and honestly; however, it does require that palliative care nurses and other clinicians communicate skillfully in ways that assist patients and families to sustain hope. There are many articles describing empirically derived methods for delivering bad news sensitively and communicating in ways that maintain hope.[56,69]

Programs to Enhance Hopefulness

In addition to discrete actions that individual nurses take to foster hope, several investigators have developed and tested programs to enhance hope in people with life-threatening illness.

Duggleby and colleagues[26] evaluated the effectiveness of the *Living With Hope Program* (LWHP), a brief intervention designed for older adults with advanced cancer receiving home-based palliative care services. Grounded in their earlier research,[46] the LWHP is a 1-week intervention consisting of a visit from a trained assistant, a copy of the film "Living With Hope," and a choice of one of three hope-focused activities. The investigators found that compared to the control group, LWHP participants reported greater hope and existential quality of life 1 week following the intervention. The LWHP also has been pilot-tested in a sample of 10 family caregivers, and results suggest that the program may increase hope and quality of life in this group.[70]

Rustoen and colleagues[29] studied the effects of a professional-led group intervention on hope and psychological distress in a community-based sample of cancer patients. The intervention consisted of eight 2-hour sessions focused on belief in oneself and in one's ability, emotional reactions, relationships with others, active involvement, spiritual beliefs and values, and acknowledgment that there is a future. The results showed increased hope levels and decreased psychological distress immediately following the intervention; however, it was not sustained at the 3- and 12-month assessments. The investigators suggested that like other cognitive-behavioral interventions, additional "booster sessions" would have been helpful.

Ensuring the Self-Knowledge Necessary to Provide Palliative Care

Providing holistic palliative care requires a broad range of skills. Astute management of physical symptoms and a solid command of technical skills must be matched with an ability to provide psychosocial and spiritual care for patients and families at a time of great vulnerability. To nurture these latter skills, nurses should continually reflect on and evaluate their own hopes, beliefs, and biases and identify how these factors influence their care. In an intriguing study, investigators examined the relationship between nurses' hope and their comfort in caring for and communicating with dying children and their families. They found that, after controlling for number of years in nursing, nurses' hope and hours of palliative care education both were significantly associated with comfort in caring for dying children and their families.[71] These findings underscore the importance of education as well as self-reflection in delivering compassionate, skilled palliative care. In providing high-quality care, nurses also should evaluate how they are affected by patients' and families' responses and strategies to maintain hope. For example, does it anger or frustrate the nurse that the patient seems to refuse to acknowledge that his or her disease is incurable? Is this anger communicated nonverbally or verbally to the patient or family? In addition to self-reflection, it is important for palliative care nurses to remain hopeful while working with dying patients by engaging in self-care activities.

Summary

Hope is central to the human experience of living and dying, and it is integrally entwined with spiritual and psychosocial well-being. Although terminal illness can challenge and even temporarily diminish hope, the dying process does not inevitably bring despair. The human spirit, manifesting its creativity and resiliency, can forge new and deeper hopes at the end of life. Palliative care nurses play important roles in supporting patients and families with this process by providing expert physical, psychosocial, and spiritual care. Sensitive, skillful attention to maintaining hope can enhance quality of life and contribute significantly to a "good death" as defined by the patient and family. Fostering hope is a primary means by which palliative care nurses accompany patients and families on the journey through terminal illness.

References

1. Feudtner C. Hope and the prospect of healing at the end of life. *J Alternative and Complementary Med.* 2005;11(1):S23–S30.
2. Fromm E. *The Revolution of Hope.* New York, NY: Bantam; 1968.
3. Marcel G. *Homo Viator: Introduction to a Metaphysic of Hope.* New York, NY: Harper & Row; 1962.
4. Menninger K. Hope. *Bulletin of the Menninger Clinic.* 1987;51(5):447–462.

5. Ersek M. Examining the process and dilemmas of reality negotiation. *Image—J of Nurs Scholarship*. 1992;24(1):19–25.

6. Snyder CR, Rand KL. The case against false hope. *Amer Psychol.* 2003;58(10):820–822; authors' reply 823–824.

7. Dufault K, Martocchio B. Hope: its spheres and dimensions. *Nurs Clin of North Am.* 1985;20:379–391.

8. De Graves S, Aranda S. Living with hope and fear—the uncertainty of childhood cancer after relapse. *Cancer Nurs.* Jul-Aug 2008;31(4):292–301.

9. Kylma J, Vehvilainen-Julkunen K, Lahdevirta J. Dynamically fluctuating hope, despair and hopelessness along the HIV/AIDS continuum as described by caregivers in voluntary organizations in Finland. *Issues in Ment Health Nurs.* 2001;22(4):353–377.

10. Kylma J, Vehvilainen-Julkunen K, Lahdevirta J. Hope, despair and hopelessness in living with HIV/AIDS: a grounded theory study. *J Adv Nurs.* 2001;33(6):764–775.

11. Morse JM, Penrod J. Linking concepts of enduring, uncertainty, suffering, and hope. *Image—J of Nurs Scholarship*. 1999;31(2):145–150.

12. Cutcliffe J, Herth K. The concept of hope in nursing 2: hope and mental health nursing. *Br J Nurs.* 2002;11(13):885–889.

13. Gibson LM. Inter-relationships among sense of coherence, hope, and spiritual perspective (inner resources) of African-American and European-American breast cancer survivors. *Appl Nurs Res.* 2003;16(4):236–244.

14. Haase JE, Britt T, Coward DD, Leidy NK, Penn PE. Simultaneous concept analysis of spiritual perspective, hope, acceptance and self-transcendence. *Image—J Nurs Scholarship*. 1992;24(2):141–147.

15. Herth KA. The relationship between level of hope and level of coping response and other variables in patients with cancer. *Oncol Nurs Forum.* 1989;16(1):67–72.

16. Carson V, Soeken KL, Shanty J, Terry L. Hope and spiritual well-being: essentials for living with AIDS. *Perspect Psychiatr Care.* 1990;26(2):28–34.

17. Fehring RJ, Miller JF, Shaw C. Spiritual well-being, religiosity, hope, depression, and other mood states in elderly people coping with cancer. *Oncol Nurs Forum.* 1997;24(4):663–671.

18. Duggleby W, Wright K. Transforming hope: how elderly palliative patients live with hope. *Can J Nurs Res.* 2005;37(2):70–84.

19. Fanos JH, Gelinas DF, Foster RS, Postone N, Miller RG. Hope in palliative care: from narcissism to self-transcendence in amytrophic lateral sclerosis *J Palliat Med.* 2008;11(3):470–475.

20. Borneman T, Brown-Saltzman K. Meaning in illness. In: Ferrell BR, Coyle N, eds. *Oxford Textbook of Palliative Nursing.* 3rd ed. New York, NY: Oxford University Press; 2010:673–683.

21. Harris GE, Larsen D. HIV peer counseling and the development of hope: perspectives from peer counselors and peer counseling recipients. *AIDS Patient Care and STDs.* 2007;21(11):843–860.

22. Kavradim ST, Ozer ZC, Bozcuk H. Hope in people with cancer: a multivariate analysis from Turkey. *J Adv Nurs.* 2013;69(5):1183–1196.

23. Mattioli JL, Repinski R, Chappy SL. The meaning of hope and social support in patients receiving chemotherapy. *Oncol Nursing Forum.* 2008;35(5):822–829.

24. Cotter VT. Hope in early-stage dementia: a concept analysis. *Holistic Nurs Pract.* 2009;23(5):297–301.

25. Reinke LF, Shannon SE, Engelberg RA, Young JP, Curtis JR. Supporting hope and prognostic information: nurses' perspectives on their role when patients have life-limiting prognoses. *J Pain Symptom Manage.* 2010;39(6):982–992.

26. Duggleby WD, Degner L, Williams A, et al. Living with hope: initial evaluation of a psychosocial hope intervention for older palliative home care patients. *J Pain Symptom Manage.* 2007;33(3):247–257.

27. Weis RS, Speridakos EC. A meta-analysis of hope enhancement strategies in clinical and community settings. *Psychol of Well-Being: Theory Res Pract.* 2011;1(5):1–16.

28. Kylma J, Duggleby W, Cooper D, Molander G. Hope in palliative care: an integrative review. *Palliat Supportive Care.* 2009;7(3):365–377.

29. Rustoen T, Cooper BA, Miaskowski C. A longitudinal study of the effects of a hope intervention on levels of hope and psychological distress in a community-based sample of oncology patients. *Eur J Oncol Nurs.* 2011;15(4):351–357.

30. Lazarus RS, Folkman S. *Stress, Appraisal, and Coping.* New York, NY: Springer; 1984.

31. Folkman S. Stress, coping, and hope. *Psycho-oncology.* 2010;19(9):901–908.

32. Rustoen T, Cooper BA, Miaskowski C. The importance of hope as a mediator of psychological distress and life satisfaction in a community sample of cancer patients. *Cancer Nurs.* 2010;33(4):258–267.

33. Olsson L, Ostlund G, Strang P, Jeppsson Grassman E, Friedrichsen M. Maintaining hope when close to death: insight from cancer patients in palliative home care. *Int J Palliat Nurs.* 2010;16(12):607–612.

34. Rawdin B, Evans C, Rabow MW. The relationships among hope, pain, psychological distress, and spiritual well-being in oncology outpatients. *J Palliat Med.* 2013;16(2):167–172.

35. Zhang Y, Law CK, Yip PSF. Psychological factors associated with the incidence and persistence of suicidal ideation. *J Affective Disord.* 2011;133(3):584–590.

36. Joiner TE Jr, Brown JS, Wingate LR. The psychology and neurobiology of suicidal behavior. *Ann Rev Psych.* 2005;56:287–314.

37. Dees MK, Vernooij-Dassen MJ, Dekkers WJ, Vissers KC, van Weel C. "Unbearable suffering": a qualitative study on the perspectives of patients who request assistance in dying. *J Med Ethics.* 2011;37(12):727–734.

38. Phuong Do D, Dowd JB, Ranjit N, House, JS, Kaplan, GA. Hopelessness, depression, and early markers of endothelial dysfunction in U.S. adults. *Psychosom Med.* 2010;72(7):613–619.

39. Kylma J, Juvakka T. Hope in parents of adolescents with cancer—factors endangering and engendering parental hope. *Euro J Oncol Nurs.* 2007;11(3):262–271.

40. Salmon P, Hill J, Ward J, Gravenhorst K, Eden T, Young B. Faith and protection: the construction of hope by parents of children with leukemia and their oncologists. *The Oncologist.* 2012;17(3):398–404.

41. Mack JW, Wolfe J, Cook EF, Grier HE, Cleary PD, Weeks JC. Hope and prognostic disclosure. *J Clin Oncol.* 2007;25(35):5636–5642.

42. Hirsch JK, Sirois FM, Lyness JM. Functional impairment and depressive symptoms in older adults: Mitigating effects of hope. *Br J Health Psychol.* 2011;16(4):744–760.

43. Duggleby W, Hicks D, Nekolaichuk C, et al. Hope, older adults, and chronic illness: A metasynthesis of qualitative research. *J Adv Nurs.* 2012;68(6):1211–1223.

44. Moore SL. The experience of hope and aging: a hermeneutic photography study. *J Gerontol Nurs.* 2012;38(10):28–36.

45. Esbensen BA, Swane CE, Hallberg IR, Thome B. Being given a cancer diagnosis in old age: a phenomenological study. *Int J Nurs Stud.* 2008;45(3):393–405.

46. Duggleby W, Wright K. Transforming hope: how elderly palliative patients live with hope. *Can J Nurs Res.* 2005;37(2):70–84.

47. Duggleby W, Williams A, Wright K, Bollinger S. Renewing everyday hope: the hope experience of family caregivers of persons with dementia. *Issues in Ment Health Nurs.* 2009;30(8):514–521.

48. Holtslander LF, Duggleby WD. The hope experience of older bereaved women who cared for a spouse with terminal cancer. *Qualitative Health Res.* 2009;19(3):388–400.

49. Holtslander LF, Duggleby W, Williams AM, Wright KE. The experience of hope for informal caregivers of palliative patients. *J Palliat Care.* 2005;21(4):285–291.

50. Lohne V, Miaskowski C, Rustoen T. The relationship between hope and caregiver strain in family caregivers of patients with advanced cancer. *Cancer Nurs.* 2012;35(2):99–105.

51. Duggleby WD, Swindle J, Peacock S, Ghosh S. A mixed methods study of hope, transitions, and quality of life in family caregivers of persons with Alzheimer's disease. *BMC Geriatrics.* 2011;11:88.

52. Eliott JA, Olver IN. Hope and hoping in the talk of dying cancer patients. *Social Sci Med.* 2007;64(1):138–149.

53. Eliott JA, Olver IN. Hope, life, and death: a qualitative analysis of dying cancer patients' talk about hope. *Death Stud.* 2009;33(7):609–638.

54. Buckley J, Herth K. Fostering hope in terminally ill patients. *Nurs Standard.* 2004;19(10):33–41.

55. Shinn EH, Taylor CL, Kilgore K, et al. Associations with worry about dying and hopelessness in ambulatory ovarian cancer patients. *Palliat Supportive Care.* 2009;7(3):299–306.

56. Curtis JR, Engelberg R, Young JP, et al. An approach to understanding the interaction of hope and desire for explicit prognostic information among individuals with severe chronic obstructive pulmonary disease or advanced cancer. *J Palliat Med.* 2008;11(4):610–620.

57. Berendes D, Keefe FJ, Somers TJ, Kothadia SM, Porter LS, Cheavens JS. Hope in the context of lung cancer: relationships of hope to symptoms and psychological distress. *J Pain Symptom Manage.* 2010;40(2):174–182.

58. Farone DW, Fitzpatrick TR, Bushfield SY. Hope, locus of control, and quality of health among elder Latina cancer survivors. *Soc Work Health Care* 2008;46(2):51–70.

59. Purnell LD. The Purnell Model for cultural competence. In: Purnell LD, ed. *Transcultural Health Care: A Culturally Competent Approach.* 4th ed. Philadelphia, PA: F. A. Davis; 2013:15–44.

60. Beauchamp TL, Childress JF. *Principles of Biomedical Ethics.* 7th ed. New York, NY: Oxford University Press; 2013.

61. Oliffe J, Thorne S, Hislop TG, Armstrong EA. "Truth telling" and cultural assumptions in an era of informed consent. *Fam Community Health.* 2007;30(1):5–15.

62. Shaw S. Exploring the concepts behind truth-telling in palliative care. *Int J Palliat Nurs*. 2008;14(7):356–359.

63. Giger JN, Davidhizar RE, Fordham P. Multi-cultural and multi-ethnic considerations and advanced directives: developing cultural competency. *J Cult Diversity*. 2006;13(1):3–9.

64. Olsman E, Leget C, Onwuteaka-Philipsen B, Willems D. Should palliative care patients' hope be truthful, helpful or valuable? An interpretative synthesis of literature describing healthcare professionals' perspectives on hope of palliative care patients. *Palliat Med*. 2014;28(1):59–70.

65. Farran CJ, Wilken C, Popovich JM. Clinical assessment of hope. *Issues Ment Health Nurs*. 1992;13(2):129–138.

66. Holtslander L, Duggleby W. An inner struggle for hope: insights from the diaries of bereaved family caregivers. *Int J Palliat Nurs*. 2008;14(10):478–484.

67. Holtslander LF. Caring for bereaved family caregivers: analyzing the context of care. *Clin J Oncol Nurs*. 2008;12(3):501–506.

68. Farran CJ, Herth KA, Popovich JM. *Hope and Hopelessness: Critical Clinical Constructs*. Thousand Oaks, CA: SAGE; 1995.

69. Robinson CA. "Our best hope is a cure." Hope in the context of advance care planning. *Palliat Supportive Care*. 2012:1–8.

70. Duggleby W, Wright K, Williams A, Degner L, Cammer A, Holtslander L. Developing a Living With Hope program for caregivers of family members with advanced cancer. *J Palliat Care*. 2007;23(1):24–31.

71. Feudtner C, Santucci G, Feinstein JA, Snyder CR, Rourke MT, Kang TI. Hopeful thinking and level of comfort regarding providing pediatric palliative care: a survey of hospital nurses. *Pediatrics*. 2007;119(1):e186–e192.

Index